COMMITMENT TO FITNESS:
REAL FITNESS FOR REAL PEOPLE

COMMITMENT TO FITNESS: REAL FITNESS FOR REAL PEOPLE

▼

Dr. David Lemberg, D.C.

Writers Club Press
San Jose New York Lincoln Shanghai

Commitment to Fitness:
Real Fitness for Real People

Writers Club Press
an imprint of iUniverse.com, Inc.

For information address:
iUniverse.com, Inc.
5220 S 16th, Ste. 200
Lincoln, NE 68512
www.iuniverse.com

ISBN: 0-595-15134-5

Printed in the United States of America

To my father,
Herman Louis Lemberg,

my mother,
Anita Lemberg Fenson,

and my stepfather,
Harry Fenson

CONTENTS

▼

A Note to My Readers

▼

I've been a fitness person all my life. I played Little League baseball as a kid, ran track in junior high school, and began studying dance—ballet, jazz, and modern—in college. I danced professionally, taught jazz dance, and later enrolled in chiropractic school. I've been in private practice in Manhattan for almost twenty years, treating a wide range of sports-related injuries. I know the human body. I know exercise. I have more than thirty years of front-line experience to share.

You may already be a fitness person, you may want to become one, or you may be experiencing some physical problems which might be helped with exercise and nutritional recommendations. Whatever your current fitness status, *Commitment to Fitness: Real Fitness for Real People* was written with you in mind.

My goal has been to write *more* than a fitness book—many excellent how-to guides are already available. I wanted to write a special fitness book, one about people, one that meets your specific needs. A book that covered *all* the basics and then went beyond, from posture and stretching, through weight-training, aerobics, and nutrition, through recovering from injury, establishing a powerful doctor–patient partnership, and coming back even stronger. Above all, a book that was life-affirming.

"Coming back stronger" is a theme running through *Commitment to Fitness*. Injury, even illness, can be an opportunity. Stuff happens to all of us. How will we respond? I've attempted to present courses of action that each of us can follow, based on easy-to-understand principles that work.

The great thing about fitness is that it's never too late to start. In fact, whatever your age, whatever shape you're in, you can improve your health and well-being. My book offers expert guidance and assistance along this life-long path.

ACKNOWLEDGEMENTS

▼

My life has been blessed with brilliant teachers. My high school English teachers, Miss Isabel Kliegman, Mr. Seymone J.D. Pansick, and Miss Deborah Tannenbaum, taught me how to think, how to get the most from my reading, and how to write with purpose.

My dance teachers molded me not only as an athlete, but as a person. Each one demanded dedication, concentration, growth. They each saw things in me that I could not see myself, and they were the shining examples of what I could become. Daily, through the years, I am informed by their timely teachings, whether I'm walking down the street, lifting weights in the gym, running in Central Park, or working with my patients. Don Farnworth was my ballet teacher. Lynn Simonson, Fred Benjamin, and Betsy Haug were my jazz dance teachers. Jimmy Truitte, Thelma Hill, and Viola Farber were my modern dance teachers. This remarkable group of individuals helped me achieve all that I've achieved.

My hands-on training as a chiropractor was provided by two mentors, Dr. Pasquale Cerasoli and Dr. Stanley Alpert. Their skill and expertise are surpassed only by their compassion. Dr. Lowell Bower, my first postgraduate instructor in chiropractic orthopedics, taught the importance of differential diagnosis. He trained his students to think "outside the box". My practice benefits every day from the teachings of these doctors.

I began weight-training in 1984 at my local YMHA. A year or so later I joined a bigger, more well-equipped gym in Manhattan, and met Ben Velazquez, one of the gym's instructors. A competitive bodybuilder, Ben was always gracious and generous with his time and expertise. He provided a solid foundation, grounded in the fundamentals, and helped me recover from numerous injuries. Each time I came back stronger.

A doctor's patients are his teachers. While I was helping them to heal, they were helping me to learn.

Finally, my thanks to Eurydice Kelley, the model for the photographs used in *Commitment to Fitness.*

Chapter 1

▼

In Search of Sound Minds and Sound Bodies

The longer I have been in practice, the more I have become convinced that people's diseases are not random occurrences. If you're sick, there is probably *something* in your life that is unacceptable to you, there is some problem or problems, some disturbance in the functioning of your family or workplace, some dissatisfaction or upset that breaks the continuity or order of your existence. Something shouldn't be.

I remember one winter, years ago, when I was having major financial challenges. I had a lot of debt, of my own making, and was very upset. During this time I developed a herpes zoster infection, described as a moderate case by my dermatologist. I learned from him that herpes zoster, or adult chickenpox, is fairly common, affecting one in ten adults. If you've had chickenpox as a child, the virus persists in a dormant state for the rest of your life, residing in the cells of the spinal cord. In ten percent of adults, the virus becomes active for a time, creating the severe pain and rash of "shingles", as the disorder is commonly called. I felt pretty bad, took antiviral medication, bathed the rashes, and recovered after four weeks or so. As I recovered, I began to question how I became ill, and what the circumstances might have been that caused the disease. If this virus is present in all those who have had chickenpox, why does it only become active in ten percent? What differentiates those who develop shingles from those who don't?

I strongly suspected that my high levels of stress were implicated, in particular, my nonstop worry, anger, and anxiety. Previously I had been well; now there were these circumstances and I succumbed to an infection. Interestingly, shingles is an infection of the nervous system; I had been pretty "nervous" about my monetary concerns. I concluded that a relationship existed between my mental state and my physical well-being. Now, of course, this conclusion is not earthshaking, but I had been able to use myself as a laboratory and I was pretty confident of my hypothesis. I proposed to myself that many illnesses were stress-related. The arena in which I could evaluate this concept was my office, where I treated people's musculoskeletal conditions and disorders.

I began to actively consider my patients' complaints and injuries in a broader context. I took on the notion that even strains and sprains were not isolated events, but rather occurred in the overall context of the person's *life*. The person's lifestyle became an important part of history taking: What type of exercise do you do? Has there been any recent change in your work or family circumstances? Have you started a new project recently? Other aspects and events became relevant in addition to the person's medical history and the circumstances of the injury or chronic complaint.

Now, I'm not looking for the *cause* of the person's pain pattern. I'm not suggesting that this *life situation* is what is causing a person's pain or disease. Rather, I'm suggesting that if something is *off* in my life or your life, if there is something unresolved that is nagging at me, something or someone I am avoiding dealing with, some concern from the past that keeps butting in on the present, then these *incomplete* situations may be implicated in the development of the illness. This is a hypothesis, of course, but it is one that can provide real benefit for the person who considers it and looks, really looks, at his life.

I'm not talking about basic wear and tear. Systems fail and things break down. However, why is it that some people can be mostly well and productive into their eighties and even nineties, and others are unfortunately dead before age fifty? Recently, a patient told me of his friend who died of a heart attack at age forty-eight. The wife of a friend of mine had lupus erythematosus and died when she was thirty-seven. My father died when he was sixty of rectal carcinoma. We all have had friends and relations who died when they were young. There are genetic predispositions, of course, inherited weaknesses or tendencies that manifest as debilitating or fatal disease. But what else might be going on here?

Is it possible that there is no real separation, no useful distinction, between the mind and the body? Is it possible that whatever occurs in your thoughts is associated on a one-to-one basis with a physiologic response? I'm not proposing anything new here. The "mind-body connection" has been described and discussed at great length elsewhere. I am proposing there are practical benefits from inquiring into this possible relationship, not as some "airy-fairy" or "woo-woo" stuff, but as something that can be of use to us, making our bodies fitter and healthier and our lives richer as a result.

This is a good place to share some things about my father. My dad died when he was young, at sixty, and I've always felt that stress had a lot to do with that. My parents divorced when I was a teenager and my father married two more times after that. He was in the Army Air Force in World War II, the radioman in planes that flew missions over Italy. He was a teamster after the war, then a salesman, and finally received his college degree in his middle forties and became an industrial arts teacher. When he died he was Dean of Students at a junior high school outside New York City. My parents were "leftists" when I was a child, engaged in workers' rights activities and the civil rights movement.

When I was fourteen years old, I attended the March on Washington in 1963 and heard Martin Luther King, Jr. deliver his "I have a dream" speech, thanks to my dad asking me to go with him on that march. When I was about ten my dad was placed in the hospital because he had chest pains. He was diagnosed as having had a "heart attack" and from that day forward he was concerned with his heart. He became a person who had had a heart attack, and for a long time he weakened noticeably. It took years for him to return to his usual lively, outgoing way of being. Much later, updated EKGs showed that there had been no damage to my father's heart. My dad became much more active after this and began to exercise again.

Looking back, my father's chest pains occurred at a time of great stress: he was changing jobs *again* and he and my mom were having many loud disagreements. Later, when he developed cancer, it seemed as if he was at the end of a long, hard road. He had become successful and satisfied in his career as an educator after years of employment in a wide variety of make-do jobs. He was on his third "family"; both his second and third wives had children of their own with their attendant demands and problems. It's my sense that his many struggles took a great toll on him and exerted a cumulative weakening effect. Cancer developed in him opportunistically, the abnormal cells flourishing in a depleted internal environment. He never did well after the initial diagnosis, the pain levels never receded for more than a day or two, and about eighteen months into treatment he simply let go and died.

I say that my father's severe illness was directly associated with his life experiences. His personal difficulties eventually wore him down. My friend Joanne died when she was forty of complications of breast cancer. She was a talented artist with a national reputation whose family life was painful and troublesome. Another friend recently died of lymphoma at age fifty-three. She had a brilliant career, but her personal life was tragic. She died within months of the initial diagnosis.

What's occurring in your life? What's missing? Are you taking on the weight of the world, as my father and my two friends did? Are you continually reviewing past events that didn't go your way, berating yourself with the supposed failures, the relationships that fell apart, the great job that you never quite seemed to get, the satisfaction that just didn't seem to come despite having a successful career? If so, welcome to the human race. But there is a price that is paid for continually making ourselves wrong, for judging and assessing ourselves, generally in the worst possible light. Human beings love to be right, and the flip side of that is making others, or situations, or ourselves wrong. It's an automatic mechanism, part of the machinery of being human. In the context of being well, I suggest there is a physiologic response to this ongoing judging and assessing.

I used to have a lot of lower back pain. Yes, I'll admit it. These problems started in a typical fashion, when I was twenty, helping a friend move from one apartment to another. I bent over to pick up a stereo speaker and—bang—I couldn't straighten up and spent the next five days on bed rest. I had problems for years afterward, even developing sciatica in my left leg that persisted for months. In my first career, I was a professional dancer. (More on this later.) Every so often my back would "go out" in dance class and I would be out for a week. When this happened during a rehearsal period or a series of performances I would just have to keep going. I danced a lot in pretty bad pain. Eventually I started chiropractic treatment and the spasms resolved.

That was twenty-five years ago. Seven or eight years ago I developed chronic, daily lower back pain. And, being stoic, I just lived with it. Dancers develop a high pain threshold. I was used to pain, having danced, and I simply tolerated this back pain. Also, in a connected pattern, whenever I took a car trip I would develop neck and upper back pain after about an hour of driving. I would be very uncomfortable in my car and began to avoid trips that lasted more than two hours. I thought this was just how things were: I would go driving and after an hour have pain for the rest of the trip. Not much fun.

Interestingly, about a year or so ago, both the back and neck pain went away. I rarely have back pain now. What was the difference? One major difference is that I stopped, to a great extent, judging and assessing people. You've heard the joke about the guy driving a car: Everybody driving slower than him is an *idiot;* everybody driving faster than him is a *maniac.* That's how I was behind the wheel. Everyone else was an idiot or a maniac. I was the only competent driver on the road. Looking back on all those years, I can say that I was in a continual state of upset while driving. I was angry and tense. Everything was wrong. People cut you off. They drift into your lane. They're too slow. They're too fast. They don't let you change lanes. There's too much traffic. There's too much construction. How come they're in *my way?* Apparently, after about an hour of this internal conversation my upper back muscles would get so tense that I would experience pain, pain that worsened for the duration of the trip. Not much possibility for a peaceful, enjoyable ride.

I saw that I lived like that during the day, too. This is how I would be, walking down the street: What's with all these potholes! Why did that person look at me that way? What do you mean, bumping into me? Don't blow smoke right in my face! What's with all the noise? (Remember, this is New York City!) Stop that honking! That bicycle almost ran me over! Jackhammers, ambulances, sirens, yelling, pushing! This is how I experienced a stroll in Manhattan. Everything was wrong. No wonder I had back pain!

I began to notice my behavior, becoming aware of these habitual thought patterns and physiologic responses. Of course, even though I've increased my self-awareness, old mechanisms can reassert themselves. A few months ago I received a call from a telecommunications company, to check on the status of a presumably overdue account. I had ordered a pager, didn't use it, and returned it. The company continued to send me bills, despite my having called to confirm their receipt of the pager. So instead of managing the conversation with the collections representative, working it out peacefully, I went to war with him.

I was sarcastic, argumentative, confrontational. My heart was pounding and I could feel my back tightening up, getting more tight and even painful with each parry and thrust. I asked for the name of his supervisor and told him I would be writing a letter. Truly I was the customer from hell. I observed myself doing this, stupefied by my performance, yet continued to indulge myself. I made this customer rep and his company completely wrong, and justified myself and my position. I won the conversation, but lost my self-possession. And I paid a heavy price—I had back pain for the first time in more than a year, and it lasted for weeks. I had experienced no physical trauma—I wasn't in a fight, hadn't tripped and fallen, didn't lift a heavy weight—but my back was in spasm and I had daily pain. So there was a one-to-one relationship between stress—an upset—and physical pain. I had never experienced this association so dramatically.

I concluded there was an exact connection between my mental state and my physical functioning. I experienced back pain, whether upper or lower or both, whenever I was upset, angry, annoyed, thwarted, or challenged. If I let go of being upset, my pain went away. I became more finely attuned to this relationship. If I was walking down Broadway and I experienced an upset, regarding either a person or a circumstance, boom! Back pain. I began to inquire into this association with my chiropractic patients.

Using an anecdotal, conversational approach, rather than a reproducible method utilizing questionnaires and statistics, I hypothesized that a strong association exists between a person's physical pain or disease and their self-image and life circumstances. I don't mean to be banal here, nor do I intend to be simplistic. It is my experience, however, that pain and disease do not just happen. Disease and pain are not random events, however random they may appear. I propose that physical functioning breaks down in the presence of ongoing threats to one's sense of self, ongoing threats to one's sense of survival. These threats may be real or imagined; it is one's perception that drives the process.

I am suggesting there exists a profound mind-body connection. What goes on in the mind is reflected in the body; what occurs in the body is reflected in the mind. None of this is new; we've been hearing these kinds of statements for years and many books have been written on this theme. What may be new is the concept of "access". Given a mind/body connection, how can we develop access to health and well-being? I propose this access is available through the physical realm, via consistent, enjoyable exercise and fitness activities. We'll look at, in depth, a variety of these activities and their comprehensive benefits, and investigate how each of us can incorporate fitness into a well-rounded, busy life. Let's get started.

CHAPTER 2

▼

I CAME. I SAW.
I WORKED-OUT.

The world of exercise is wide and wonderful and includes activities ranging from brisk walking to snow skiing. I'll admit I'm a bit biased in that I have been involved in sports and other exercise stuff since I was a child. I started in Little League at age eight and played until I was twelve. I ran track in junior high school; I wasn't on any teams in high school but participated in President Kennedy's physical fitness program for young Americans. We did sit-ups and pull-ups, climbed ropes, did elementary routines on the parallel bars and the horse, played basketball and volleyball, lifted weights, and had a generally great time. I started taking dance classes in college, beginning with elementary modern dance classes in the Lester Horton technique and progressing to jazz dance and ballet classes. I developed into a good dancer and was fortunate to obtain my union card, performing in summer stock and with dance companies in

New York City. After leaving the dance field I started lifting weights for exercise, did that for many years, and started running about ten years ago.

So I've been exercising in some way, relatively consistently, and with good intensity, for more than thirty years. I have some expertise. In fact, to be totally accurate, exercise is a way of life for me. It is an important part of who I am and how I function in the world. Exercise is an integral part of my health and well-being. I intentionally bring this to my private practice of chiropractic. If you aren't already exercising consistently when you begin as a patient in my office, you'll probably start as soon as you're able. As I've said, in my office, exercise is an integral component of getting well.

OK, let's look at a few things. For many people, the possibility of exercising brings up all kinds of memories and associations, not all of them empowering. Some of these internal conversations might be "I'm overweight"; "I haven't exercised in years"; "I don't have the time"; "I'm too old"; "I don't like to exercise"; "I'm fine the way I am"; "I'm embarrassed to go to the gym"; and so on. With these conversations in the background, there's no way that anyone will start exercising if they are *told* to do it. I know you won't start training just because I said so, just because I *recommended* it.

The will to begin comes from you, the person who will be the one working up the sweat. It's your choice, and ultimately you're the only one who can make this choice. Let's put a few questions on the table. One question is, "What type of exercise would you like to do?" There are many types of exercise, all of them possessing particular value. In general, exercise that has an aerobic quality packs the most punch, provides the most overall benefit. (We're not looking to train body-builders here. As we'll see, weight training is a key component of a well-designed fitness program.) Aerobic exercise includes the following:

- Aerobic exercise classes
- Running
- Brisk walking

- Bicycle machines or brisk cycling
- Stair-climbing machines

Other repetitive exercises, such as swimming or rowing, can become aerobic if they are done rapidly enough. Later on we'll discuss the concept of *target zone,* the range of heart rates at which aerobic exercise becomes efficient.

Which form of aerobics will you actually choose? The particular type doesn't matter, making the choice and beginning the program does. Select one that you think will be fun and that you will actually do. You can mix and match, or start one type and switch to another. Exercise is work, and it can also be fun.

People are funny about exercise; they know they *should* be doing it and feel guilty if they don't, or haven't in a long time. When I ask a person what type of exercise he is doing, often he will say, "Oh, I walk a lot" or "I work out at the gym three times a week". But it turns out that the walking is simply walking to work and back, not walking specifically for exercise, or the gym workouts only started two weeks ago. Let's tell the truth about exercise: most of us are not doing it, we know we should, we may even want to and regret the fact that we're not, and we simply don't know how to begin.

Here's how to begin: pick the form of aerobic activity that you think you might enjoy and start doing it. Start today, do some, not too much, and do some more tomorrow. Then wait a day and do some the next day. Like that. Keep going and soon it will become a routine. Now it's not quite that straightforward. You'll want to quit. Other things will look like they're more important or more urgent than your planned exercise. But if you do what you said you'd do, you'll experience a great sense of accomplishment. Besides that, exercise actually *feels good,* or at least it does after you have gained some familiarity with that form of exercise. Doing the exercise that you'd planned places a brick in the foundation of your fitness program.

It's interesting. The more you do the more you want to do. My stepfather recently had a third cardiac surgery. Previously he had not been a fitness poster boy. He might go walking once or twice a week, or he might not. He was almost cynical about exercise, poking gentle fun at his two stepsons who are exercise focused. Part of his postoperative routine this time was programmed physical activity. He walked around the nurses' station. He rode an exercise bike while wearing a heart monitor. Later on he graduated to using a stair-climber and walked on an inclined treadmill. He began to walk up and down his hospital corridor, which extended the length of a city block. He concluded that this physical work contributed significantly to his good recovery. He now exercises regularly, to my delight and amazement. He wants to exercise, is proud of it, looks forward to getting out there and doing it.

Your body begins to crave exercise, even after doing some for only a few days. Our bodies were designed for hard physical work; we don't do too much of this any more. Most of us don't hunt; neither do we gather. Exercise awakens these dormant systems and initiates a cascade of responses. You begin drinking more water. You fall asleep much more easily and sleep more deeply and well. Instinctively you begin to eat better: food low in nutritive content becomes less appealing; you become drawn to things like fresh fruit and multigrain breads. Your eyes gain sparkle and your skin acquires sheen. You actually stand taller.

(Anatomical note: The intervertebral discs (shock-absorbing connective tissue interposed between adjacent vertebras) account for twenty-five percent of the length of the spine. They are largely composed of water which travels into and out of the discs on a pressure gradient. If there's not much motion happening, there is a relative loss of water content and the discs lose height over the course of a day. Exercise restores this pressure gradient and the discs increase in height. So you might gain one-quarter of an inch or so, as a result of the day's exercise.) Your step is livelier, because you are that much more *alive*. You are using your body in a manner that is familiar to *it*, even though the activity may be rather unfamiliar to *you*.

Start gradually. This requires some patience. The great thing about exercise is that it's never too late to begin; on the other hand, becoming fit is definitely a process and certain facts about that process need to be honored. One fact is that your body needs to adapt to the new demands that are being placed upon it. Those of us who lift weights or run have all had training injuries. Rarely, an injury may be unavoidable, it just happens. However, the vast majority of training injuries can be avoided; they result from doing too much, doing something too soon, or poor technique. We'll talk about technique elsewhere; here I'll suggest that too much/too soon is a main culprit.

My first hamstring injury occurred in a dance class shortly after I had done my first split. I was totally psyched; *I could do a split!* So I got cocky, and even though it was only mid-spring and the weather was still cool, I jerked myself down the last quarter-inch into a full split on a day when the split just wasn't there. *Bang!* That was the sound my hamstring made as it snapped off it's origin on the base of my pelvis. That injury took almost one year to completely heal. My other two hamstring tears resulted from showing off while going across the floor in jazz dance class, trying to get extra height on a forward leg kick, trying to look good for some new young woman in the class. *Doing too much.* Ouch.

So let's say you used to be athletic when you were younger, you remember the power, the speed, and the agility you had then, or you never really exercised before but you simply want to get it going, *right now.* And you join a gym and go around with the trainer, doing a light workout. You see everybody else sweating and grunting, lifting some impressive weight, and you think, "I can do that". So the next time you go, you don't start small because you don't want them to think you *are* small, you lift too much, and strain some muscle/tendon unit. Now you've got to wait two or three weeks before you can start over. Not a great beginning.

Or you choose to start running and haven't done any lately. Possibly you never ran, it's a new type of training. You lightly jog for fifteen minutes, you feel good, and go for fifteen more. The next day your hamstrings and calves are very sore and you can't run again for ten days. Or you go out and run fast because if you are running for exercise, you should *run*. The next day you have pain in your foot or shin and you can't run again for two weeks. In fact, in either scenario you may never run again because "running is not good for me".

OK. My point is that training effectively takes time. The early stages may be slow-going, especially to those of us who are competitive, who want to see the results *now*. But the results are happening, and each time you train you are able to do more. You can run a little further, run a little faster, climb the stairs machine at a higher level, lift a few more repetitions, lift a little heavier weight. It's a gradual experience, and you can love the progressive nature of the process.

Let's look at what exercise provides for a person. First, done correctly, exercise is fun and feels good. Now, some of us are relatively deconditioned, that is, overweight and/or haven't exercised in a *really* long time. For this group, exercising may not be so much fun nor feel so good for the first few times, but I promise that it *will* be fun and feel good soon. The feeling-good part stems from many sources. You know that sense of satisfaction that comes from doing the thing you said you'd do? Each time you run, or swim, or bike you have that experience. Also, your brain produces endorphins as a response to exercise. Endorphins are neurotransmitters that enhance one's ability to tolerate pain; they are related to the opiate family. One result of increased amounts of circulating endorphins is a heightened sense of well-being—you have the experience of being alive, and present, and powerful. All this from having run for thirty minutes!

As your training continues you lose fat and gain muscle mass. Your body changes shape accordingly. Your clothes fit better. Your stomach starts to shrink. Your skin is tauter—there is less of you in places where you wished there was less and more of you in places where you hoped there would be more. Thus, another benefit of exercise is that wishing and hoping are transformed into actions and results.

We could say that exercise is a discipline. This is not saying anything rigid, fixed, or boring about exercise. The discipline part comes in the regularity, consistency, and commitment to doing the exercise. Will there be days when you don't want to do anything remotely related to exercise? Yes. Does it mean that you are a bad person, a slacker, a fitness failure if you don't? No. The key is the commitment, the intention, the choosing to exercise. Your actions will flow from your choice, your choice to be *committed* to exercising. Having chosen, you exercise regularly and consistently. Three times a week is a great place to begin. Half an hour, three times a week. Boom. You're now a person who exercises. You will begin to want to exercise, to be missing it when you're not, to be ensuring that your schedule specifically includes exercise time. Skill and mastery follow, over time. We'll be talking a lot about this.

Exercise is also like meditation. The act of meditation provides a centering and is a mechanism for renewal. Likewise with directed physical activity. The degree of concentration required to make that six-foot putt or climb that hill or swim that last two hundred yards provides something for a person. The training gained in training is applicable to other activities in one's life. You've heard about "the zone"? In sports, when you're in "the zone" you can't miss. Everything goes in, and you reach levels you never reached before.

Professional athletes are familiar with the zone. A baseball hitter will have a week in which he hits five or six home runs. Remember Reggie Jackson, in the 1978 World Series, hitting three consecutive home runs off three different pitchers? He was in the zone. Joe Montana, Michael Jordan, and Wayne Gretzky consistently achieve zone performance. I can remember one modest "zone" while shooting hoops, just shooting a basketball. I was about sixteen feet away, angled to the right of the goal, and my shots kept falling in. Swish. It was sunset, at an outdoor court in Brooklyn. The sun was going down and my shots were going in. I made nine or ten in a row. That night was years ago and my remembrance is clear and sharp. It was a peak experience.

Funny. We started talking about exercise and finished talking about life and peak experiences. Let's inquire further into this synergy as we look at the possibility of living a great life.

CHAPTER 3

▼

PREPARATION MEETS OPPORTUNITY: SELF-AWARENESS AND SELF-EXPRESSION

What's it all about anyway? Early last week, around 7 a.m. or so, I was finishing my first transcendental meditation of the day, and I was slowly opening my eyes. A thought popped into my head, one of those lightning flashes of brilliance and clarity. The thought was, *live each day as a work of art.* I caught the fleeting thought, grabbed onto it, because you know that often these moments are missed, you are not quite paying attention, and it's gone. I loved this thought, this communication from some subterranean well of wisdom and insight. *Live each day as a work of art.*

Like a masterpiece, I thought, create a masterpiece of living each day. Work at it, like a sculptor or painter, making the details as fine and beautiful as the completed project itself will be. At the end of a week, seven days, you have seven art objects, each a unique and wonderful creation.

And then, marvelously, you get to start all over again. There is no permanency in these *objets*, no concreteness. But this art has *results:* there are effects in your own life and the lives of others, possibly permanent effects. These intermingled effects are the manifestation, the *demonstration* of the art you are creating each day, caused by your intentions, attitudes, and actions. And, of course, you can make beautiful, harmonious, aesthetic art or coarse, dissonant, and ugly art. You get to choose.

I've been thinking about the days I have left. At this writing I am fifty, in my fifty-first year, and although I'm in wonderful shape you simply never know what's going to happen tomorrow. My family's long-lived, I could live into my nineties, but even if that's so I still have less than half my life left. So I've been considering that my days are numbered. Of course, I've never entertained any such thoughts up until very recently. I've done whatever I pleased, taking my time, actually *wasting* time, really not present to the finite nature of the time available to me. Not to be maudlin, but each day is a tick of the clock, and it's becoming clearer to me that I had better make each day great, starting now. I am experiencing a sense of *urgency,* and I could wonder where that urgency was before, but it doesn't matter. My experience is that I have woken up and I'm grateful for this understanding.

So I was receptive to this call to arms, to *live each day as a work of art.* The ground was prepared by my recent musings on the passage of time. I could see, if I took this on, my life would be measurably different, unrecognizable, compared to before. If I intend to live today as an artist, *an artist of life,* then there's less room for burdens, anger, or hostility. There's less room for annoyance at the little tasks that need to be managed, such as the shopping, dishes, or laundry. I could take on being *present* when doing daily routines, *choosing* to do them rather than *having* to do them, just like choosing to exercise rather than having to do it, as we discussed earlier. For example, if I'm driving somewhere I could play a game: be a great driver. Qualities inherent in a "great driver" are skill, rapid response, an intimate machine/machine interaction between driver and vehicle, the ability to visualize possible traffic situations before they develop and become problems, calmness, peacefulness, and equanimity. Whatever happens, happens. Whatever the other drivers do, I will not be stressed. Or, more realistically, I will give up the stress as soon as it occurs, rather than holding on and becoming tense and upset. I will have a great trip, regardless of the circumstances.

Preparation is required to create my road trip as a work of art. I will need to get up on time, or even early, so that I can do all the things there are to do in the morning and not be rushed. I will leave the house with time to spare, rather than allowing the absolute minimum time for the trip. My car will have been appropriately serviced (for example, there is plenty of gas in the car, the car is clean). I put out the accessories the night before (cell phone, CDs and tapes, sunglasses, fruit), not only so I don't have to scramble to find everything, but also to ensure I bring everything I want to bring. The trip is less than artistic if I've forgotten my cell phone, and am now worrying about what will happen if I need to pull over, or if I left that special CD on the coffee table. Now I'm driving and stuff happens. Slow driver in the left lane. Flash my brights; he won't move over. I start to get tense, feel my shoulders hunching, feel some neck pain, and then I remember that I'm giving up stress. OK, let it go. He's doing what he's doing, it's not personal to me. After a few minutes an opening appears and the way is clear.

Or, I'm cruising along, traffic's light, making great time, and—look out—roadside construction, big slowdown. If I've left a narrow window of time to be on time, I'm done. Here comes the tension, the muscle pain. This always happens! Can't they do this stuff at night! Come on! Let's get moving! All that anxiety, all that discomfort. Driving as art, yeah, right, tell me another! However—if I've allowed for a wider window, provided for the possibility of random events along the way, I can accept this delay for what it is: an event in my day. I may not actually *love* sitting there, stopping and going, but I will reach my destination and have fun doing it, regardless. My driving goals now are to have a great trip and minimize stress. It's so easy for me to be angry, for my heart to start pounding, to think highly unflattering thoughts about the driver who just veered into my lane. For me, these are deeply ingrained automatic mechanisms. I mean, I was an angry person for a long time. I'm learning that I actually have a choice in the matter. I can *notice* my *reaction,* and then *choose* my *response.* And who I choose to be is a great driver, experiencing the flow of events around me, skillfully charting my course toward my destination.

And, here's something else I've noticed. The more I intend to be on time, the more I am on time. (I've been living my life this way for years, now, ever since a friend observed, "If you're not early, you're late".) And, remarkably, the less stress I have about being on time, in other words, when I've prepared well and am going with the flow, the more I am just plain early. My bus gets stuck in traffic, my subway is delayed by "transit police activity" in the station ahead, but ultimately I am early. I love being on time. It's a successful outcome, which of course sets the stage for other successful outcomes, many of which I may not even have been aware were in development. That's the great thing about being on time. I did what I said I was going to do, and this is training for doing what I said I was going to do the next time.

What are some other examples of having the small, mundane, routine tasks of life come out great so that you create your day as a work of art? Well, how about going shopping and doing the laundry! In the past, these activities occurred to me as complete time wasters. Hey, I've got lots of *important* things to do! Is it really time to do the laundry again? I just did it two weeks ago! (That's a joke. Well, almost a joke.) Or, rats, I forgot to buy coffee filters. Do I have to go to the store again? Going to the supermarket used to be quite a tense experience. I would rush around the aisles, trying to do everything at once and get out of the store before the checkout lines got too long. I wouldn't take the time to make a list, believing I'd remember everything, and would usually forget to purchase some critical item, like zero-fat vegetable cooking spray or steak sauce or Half & Half. How incomplete and ineffective I'd feel, having gone shopping, something I didn't want to do in the first place, and coming home without the one thing I really needed.

Or the laundry. Who really wants to do this? Well, probably *some* people, but for me, mostly, doing the laundry has been an onerous chore, one to be delayed as long as possible, usually until it can't be postponed any longer. When I finally *have to* do it, I'm already annoyed that I've run out of stuff, can't believe I'm *wasting my time* doing the *laundry,* how trivial, how pointless, isn't there a better way, how come everybody else is in the laundry room when I'm there, why didn't I remember to buy detergent or softener, or something else critical to the task of laundry. So, something is *wrong.* There is something wrong with the whole process of laundry, or shopping, and every related event proves this so. Life should not be set up this way, where people with important things to do have to do these other, not important, things. There's no way for me to win in this. Of course, one solution would be to hire someone to shop and do laundry for me. By hiring someone, I would solve the short-term annoyance problem, but I wouldn't solve the *living* problem.

What I could do instead, and have taken on doing, is consider that life is what is happening *now.* That life is, in fact, composed of all these *now* moments, and that the most fun, the greatest self-expression, is obtained by making the moments great, making the *now* great. How exactly do you do this? Well, I think this "way of being" is a developed skill. We wouldn't just naturally say, "Oh, great, I'm doing the laundry and going shopping today". Or, "How terrific, this is the morning I'm going to the Motor Vehicles Bureau". And, interestingly, if I have taken on being great in life, somehow something is going to occur to test my resolve, giving me a clear opportunity to witness exactly where I am.

For example, I recently traveled from New York to San Diego, on December 24th, to visit my brother and his family. My ticket read "New York to San Diego", didn't indicate a connection, and I thought I had a rare direct flight to the coast. Not exactly. When I arrived at LaGuardia Airport I learned my first destination was Atlanta. All right, that's fine, I'll get where I'm going. We have an hour delay attempting to land at Atlanta-Hartsfield, and then there is an unscheduled equipment change. OK, go to another gate, rush a little. Arrive at the new gate, the connecting plane's not ready, in fact, another plane isn't available as yet. OK, get some lunch. Go back to the gate, now there's another gate change, go clear across the airport to the international concourse. Wait for the new plane to land, be serviced, and finally depart for San Diego four hours late. Total travel time, point to point, fourteen hours.

Now, I know this is not the worst air travel story. As we're driving to my brother's house, he tells me of a twenty-hour trip from San Francisco to New York. And, of course, it was only an inconvenience, not an air-travel accident. But I'm aware of how I would have *reacted* in the past. I would have been tense, angry, and annoyed, my neck and back would be tight and painful, after landing I might have strained back muscles lifting my luggage and been even more unhappy and upset. This has all happened before. So rather than being *victimized* by events, I *chose* to be *present,* to be part of events. In fact, I chose to have a good time in the face of some challenging circumstances. I spoke with and joked with a lot of people, intending for them to have the possibility of a little fun too. Not like an idiot, just sharing the experience. The terminal's food area was crowded, so I sat down at a table occupied by a seventy-ish woman, and spent a wonderful half-hour speaking with her about her life and family and my life and family. We became friendly in a brief time. That never would have happened had I been sullen and noncommunicative because my plane was delayed.

Now I'm not suggesting that one become a Pollyanna, goofily smiling and saying everything's OK when it blatantly isn't. I do suggest that one always has a choice. You can be this or that, and shift from one choice to another in a moment. Of course this takes practice and skill, both of which flow from intentionality. I can be an automatic machine reacting to the circumstances around me, buffeted by random events. I'm happy, sad, mad, upset, overjoyed, or stressed depending on my environment. In this mode,

I have no center, I'm not much different from a cork bobbing in a bathtub or a kite drifting in the wind. If I've had a busy day in my office, I'm happy; if people have canceled, if the day was slow, I'm upset. If my car is waiting for me when I go to the garage, I'm happy; if I have to wait five minutes for it to be brought up, even though I called for it, I'm annoyed.

Being like that was always uncomfortable. Since so many of life's events are random, without apparent causation, certainly with no consideration for my desires and wishes, I was in a constant state of upset. The subway is late. The subway is crowded. The bridge toll plaza is jammed. The store doesn't have my size in stock. The new appliance is defective. The movie line is so long. My clothes aren't ready at the dry cleaners. The list is endless. And, ultimately, pointless. Pointless, since, if I am (speaking of the human "I") the pinnacle of millennia of evolutionary progress and development, what does it matter if my tan slacks are a day late?

What is the access to choosing another way of being? The first step is gaining the awareness that I have a choice, that my behavior is not necessarily automatic and predetermined, that there is an opportunity to *respond* rather than *react.* If I'm reacting, then my automatic mechanisms are in charge. If I am responding, then I have a choice. And what I choose is to be *present,* in the moment, and if I'm present then my choices will be naturally authentic. My choices will be authentic expressions of who I am, rather than some automatic behavior of what I have been trained to be.

For example, I'm waiting for a taxi on Park Avenue and East Seventy-first Street, down the block from my office. It's 7 p.m. and it's raining. My learned behavior as a New Yorker would be something like this: It's raining; there are no cabs. Cab drivers are rude, they don't speak English, they're unsafe drivers, they don't care if you're in a rush. That's a lot of baggage to carry around when you're traveling by taxi. With this automatic set-up, I'm already upset before anything has happened. There's no possibility for even a bland experience, certainly no opportunity for a *pleasant* cab ride. By the time an empty cab arrives at my corner I'm all worked up; I *knew* there'd be no cabs! I don't greet the cab driver, simply climb in and bark out my destination. He senses my annoyance, my rudeness, and jumps away from the curb. I've barely settled in and am flung against the seatback, my head rocking backwards. Now I'm *really* annoyed. I *know* these guys can't drive. Well, you can see how the rest of my evening will go. Not very well. I meet the people I'm meeting, start complaining about how terrible cab service is in New York, complain about the bad weather, naturally everybody agrees with me, I succeed in having the others be anxious and upset (although I didn't *mean* to do that), and we're all uncomfortable and irritable. Could I have arrived at the meeting or party and created something other than stress and discomfort? Is It possible to have a choice here, to intervene in this cycle of automatic behavior and unpleasant experience?

Choice becomes possible after the realization that most of my behavior has been automatic. I'm operating on automatic pilot and reacting. Rainy day equals this. Cab driver equals that. With an awareness of my machine-like functioning, an opportunity exists for creating something else. A choice. How else might I have been on such an evening? Well, for starters, I could choose to be unaffected by the weather. Yes, it's raining or snowing, the wind is blowing, it's too cold or too hot, but this is still a day in my life, and as such it's too important to be thrown away on a bad mood related to "bad" weather. I've come to this place of "weather acceptance" very slowly. Long ago I lived in Amsterdam for a year, a city where the sun doesn't shine too often or for too long. It rains a lot there. It took me years to get over this. I've always "needed" the sun; I'm not happy if the sun isn't shining. After living in Holland, whenever there was a stretch of several days of clouds and rain (actually, this is not uncommon in New York) I would be pretty miserable. My state was dependent on the weather. New York winters can be cold, wet, and long. Mostly, I didn't do too well in the winter.

I used to think this was meteorology; lately I've discovered it was just me. (It was "me-teorology". Sorry.) Others have described similar states; there's even a name for this malaise: "seasonal affective disorder". I'll assert that what's needed here is less of an environmental change and more of a choice change. OK, it's raining or cloudy or whatever. Who am *I* going to be today? Is my day going to be ruled by my environment, or do I get to say how it's going to go today? I began to operate in the "I get to say" mode and to my delight, and really, surprise, my recent winters have been fun and productive. Of course, I *wish* it was sunny and warm in January, but that's called southern California, not New York. My *choosing* has made weather mostly incidental. Naturally, my old thought patterns do return, unbeckoned, in an instant, when I'm splashing through puddles or slush or when my umbrella turns inside out. And then I can choose again; there is the possibility of letting go of the habitual reaction and returning to a response: a choice.

"Letting go of the habitual reaction". Several things are required for this to occur. One is the willingness to inquire into the possibility that we function automatically most of the time. Yes, we have free will, but do we do much with this awesome power and capability? Mostly not. Mostly we are on automatic pilot. This is easily observed in New York, where large numbers of people with blank, cheerless faces can be observed on any rush-hour bus or subway. Life is routine. There's no joy, but only pain and stress and obligations and difficulty. Where's the fun, the thrill, the excitement of being alive? Gone. Gone with the repetition, the known, the familiar. Mostly we speak the language of defeat, automatic phrases of those who are beaten down by the circumstances of their lives. "I knew it wouldn't work out." "Why bother, it'll only be more of the same." "I can't wait for the holidays to be over." "Do you believe what happened to me?" "They're all a bunch of crooks." "It's no use." And so on. This is all automatic. We say these things without thinking; our parents and friends say them, and we say them, too. We hear these phrases on TV sit-coms and on news broadcasts, the media reinforcing our helplessness, automaticity, and despair.

So a first step toward "living each day as a work of art" is acknowledging our automatic machinery. Be aware of being a machine; notice the machine-like reactions and behavior. When I was a kid growing up in Brooklyn my family lived across the street from a private religious school. I went to public school and when I walked home I walked past and through large groups of the private school kids on *their* way home. It was obvious that we were different: they wore uniforms and I didn't. And, equally obviously, the reason I didn't wear a uniform was because I was of a different religion. We were kids, and nobody would get out of anybody else's way. So I would walk along, banging shoulders with the boys from the private school. Sometimes we would walk right into each other and push off, saying tough words, nobody backing down.

Walking home was difficult and sometimes scary. The goofy part was that I expected them to get out of *my way*. And, naturally, they probably expected me to get out of *their way*. So we kept ramming into each other. Now, as an adult, I walk through the streets of Manhattan expecting people to get out of my way. This is automatic behavior, except now it's even more stupid and dangerous. I've learned to notice this automatic reaction to people walking in my direction, let go of the anger and hostility that are automatically generated, and *choose another way of being,* specifically, one of politeness, care, and consideration for another. As a kid I decided it was *weak* to move out of the way. This automatic association is no longer appropriate (in retrospect it wasn't appropriate then, either). If I can recognize this behavior as automatic, then I have the opportunity to choose something else. Unrecognized, the behavior simply *runs* me, with all the consequences that can be imagined. When my behavior is automatic, unrecognized, then I am simply a machine, *reacting,* and unwelcome things happen. Awareness provides the possibility of a choice.

So the shift toward *living your life* starts with awareness. The next question is are you willing to give up these automatic behaviors? This isn't so easy. Automatic behaviors are habits, deeply ingrained, they've dug deep grooves through which the path of least resistance flows. They are familiar, comfortable, and even *natural.* By adulthood, these well-known mechanisms keep us going on the track we've laid out for ourselves, often by default. We are safe. And, yes, there is a place for automaticity. If our lower brain functions were not automatic we'd be in a lot of trouble. Do you *know* how to make your heart beat faster or slower in response to an instantaneous demand? Do you *know* how to convert salmon fillet, mashed potatoes, and broccoli into useful energy sources? Do you *know* how to walk and run? No, of course not. These processes are automatic, managed by the brainstem, cerebellum, and autonomic nervous system. I'll propose it is when our *higher* brain functions are automatic that we lose something, lose choices, lose opportunities, lose our human-ness. If I recognize this as a loss, if I'd like to see what else is possible in my life other than the "same old, same old", I might be ready to start inquiring into *what am I willing to give up?*

It's a scary question. There's a tremendous holding on to what we know, what we think we know. I've been treating a recent patient, Marjorie, for chronic neck and lower back pain. Marjorie has had these pains on and off for years; in the last few months she's been experiencing daily pain. There was nothing unusual in her history, the physical examination demonstrated musculoskeletal dysfunction, nothing more, and x-rays were unremarkable. I treated Marjorie with spinal manipulation, gave her stretches for her thighs and calves, and after a few weeks she returned to some aerobic exercise. She was doing very well, had improved about eighty percent over six weeks, and then suffered a severe worsening right after the Christmas holiday.

On the Monday morning after the Christmas weekend, Marjorie was doing hamstring stretches on the floor, and severely injured her back when she attempted to get up. She hobbled into my office, unable to stand erect, bent forward and twisted to the side. I asked her about radiating leg pain, and she described pain traveling into the fronts of both thighs. My immediate concern was that Marjorie had herniated a lumbar disc. Following a neurologic examination, I concluded she was not in immediate danger and initiated treatment for this new problem. I gave her instructions for home measures and made suggestions for appropriate medication. The next day

Marjorie was only marginally improved (she was slightly more erect), but the orthopedic signs had worsened. There were two possibilities: she had a massive, central disc herniation that was pressing on her spinal cord, or a moderate-to-severe sacroiliac joint sprain. The joint sprain could cause severe pain and radiating pain into the thighs, and would resolve with treatment within about ten days. A massive disc herniation was another matter entirely and I referred her for an immediate MRI.

I was mystified as to the cause of Marjorie's current problem. She had improved steadily and, all things being equal, should have continued to progress. A person may have minor setbacks during a course of treatment, but an acute, severe worsening would be unusual. What had occurred? We talked about what she had been doing in the last week. Yes, she had stress, and her back had been bothering her a little more before she went home for the holidays. For Marjorie, going home meant being a passenger on an eleven-hour automobile trip. While visiting, she had played with her young nephews, variously picking them up and fooling around with them on the floor. She then rode back to New York on another eleven-hour trip. None of this should have caused her *severe* pain and debility. She might have experienced increased soreness and stiffness, but nothing severe. I was at a loss to explain the event, but certain there was a hidden, undisclosed personal element.

My radiology facility called me as soon as the MRI was completed. There was a small disc herniation in the lumbar spine, an incidental finding. The radiologist said he "wouldn't even dignify it by calling it a herniation". The spinal cord and nerve roots were intact. Everything else was normal. Thus, Marjorie's symptoms were caused by a ligamentous sprain; she would be fine. Two days later, the pain in her thighs was gone, she had considerably less back pain, and was able to stand erect, although she still was moving cautiously. Marjorie was smiling again. She was making another trip to her home state that weekend, going by airplane this time. Why was she going back so soon? "Oh, I guess I didn't tell you," she said. "I have a job interview this weekend. I might be moving back there. All my family's there, and my dad will move there, too, if I take this job."

For me, this was the hidden piece of the puzzle. Marjorie's life was about to change. She has a great job in New York, her boyfriend is here, she's lived here for years. My sense is that Marjorie's recent back episode was directly related to the stress of the potential change, the worry associated with the interview, and her obligations and responsibilities to her family. She asked me, "Do you think this was caused by stress?" Yes, I do. I acknowledge this is an explanation by default, hindsight *is* 20/20, *and* there were no other causative factors. All the test results were normal. So why did it happen? Stress. There was fear, an unwillingness to move forward, to *give up*, and the outcome of this internal struggle was severe back pain.

I'm not offering these comments glibly, nor am I proposing that they are "the truth". It's not sufficient to conclude that stress is the cause of a person's pain pattern. The association is too easy and may even be dangerous, if the physician's natural suspicions are dulled by the prevalence of stress-related symptoms. Organic causes, that is, disease and pathology, must be considered and ruled out before stress can be regarded as the initiating factor. Having ruled out various significant disorders, we're left with biomechanical dysfunction as the cause of most musculoskeletal complaints.

"Biomechanical dysfunction" involves restricted joint mobility (particularly mobility of spinal joints) and irritation/inflammation of soft tissues, that is, muscle/tendon units and ligaments. Physical trauma can produce these biomechanical lesions, but in the large majority of cases I propose the initiating factor is *stress*. This is not to imply that the pain is "in your head". The pain is physical and real, there are objective, palpable, and quantifiable biomechanical consequences. What is not present is a disease. What is present is unhappiness, dissatisfaction, worry, anger, jealousy, stifled creativity, thwarted dreams, and insufficient rest. Each person can add his own brand of stress to this list. These mental states reveal themselves, directly and specifically, as physical pain. I suggest there is a one-to-one relationship between stress and biomechanical pain.

OK, I've stated the obvious. People have stress. What to do about it? The only people who don't have stress are dead. *Life* is stressful; it's a dangerous world. You don't know what's going to happen from one moment to the next. Life is highly uncertain; if events are not random they are at the least chaotic, like the weather. "Bad" things happen to "good" people; there is no "fairness doctrine". Stuff happens. If you're alive, you have stress, right? Right. So stress exists. Must there be a painful physiologic result? Possibly not. We all know at least a few people who thrive and build great lives out of some pretty stressful circumstances. For most of us, however, with our familiar, habitual ways of being, stress pretty much equals physical pain. People come to my office with all kinds of spine-related pain, radiating pain into the arms or legs, headaches, tennis elbow, knee pain, shoulder complaints, muscles spasms, and trigger points. What is the common denominator, the factor that is almost always present? Stress.

More responsibilities at work. Less responsibilities at work. Getting a new job. Leaving an old one. Starting a new love relationship. Leaving a lover. Getting married. Getting divorced. The birth of a new child. Children going off to college. Getting a cat. Getting a dog. Visiting the relatives. The relatives coming to visit. Moving to California. Moving to New York. Turning 30. Turning 40. Turning 50. Relatives die. Friends die. Gaining weight. Dieting. Buying a new car. Buying a new house. Joining a new gym. Joining a new club. Going to a party. Meeting new people. Making a speech. Being interviewed. Starting a new project. Completing an old one. Does this sound like your life? It sounds like mine, mostly. Sounds like a lot of stress. Potentially. This is it. This is life.

The factors that produce stress are myriad and complex; many people spend years in analysis or therapy, working to untangle the this and the that of their history and circumstances. This work is often necessary and appropriate. Here is another possible approach, involving inquiring into several related questions. Who am I going to be in life? Who am I going to *be* in the face of my circumstances? And then, *being that,* what am I going to do about it?

These questions imply that we have a choice. You don't have to simply roll over and take it. Also, you don't have to *be* your automatic mechanisms, either. When you're being automatic, there's no choice, and going further, no human-ness. When you're automatic, you're a machine. By noticing and then becoming aware of, or *present to,* these automatic reactions, you create a possibility of choice. My mother calls me. "Hello, David, how are you, I haven't heard from you lately. What's the matter?" Now, I love my mother. But, in the past I have easily *reacted* to her concerns, being angry or annoyed or remote and removed. With some self- awareness, however, I can observe the automatic internal reaction and intentionally choose to be something else. "Hi, Mom. Thanks for calling. I apologize for not calling you this week." No excuses, no story. Being authentic and meaning it. I've created room for us to communicate, rather than each reacting to each other from places and conversations in the distant past.

A simple, everyday example, sure. Self-awareness is a developed skill and it requires ongoing practice, in the most familiar day-to-day events. If I can be great with my mother, then I can be great with my patients, my students, and in business situations. "Being great" takes a lot of practice. Everyday there are countless situations that test my ability to be in the moment, causing myself to be great with people, despite all the things they're saying and doing and all the noise in my head. Waiting in line at the bank. Waiting in line at the post office. (Of course, a lot of this waiting will become unnecessary, with various services being automated and available online. But at some point during the day you're going to have to interact with some live bodies.) Being put on "hold" when you're calling the cable TV or telephone company.

Whenever you interact with a service person there's an opportunity for frustration and annoyance. "Why won't the cashier put the change in my hand first, instead of placing it on top of the bills so the coins slide off onto the floor!!!" Or something like that. It's an imperfect world. Things go wrong. Things break down. People make mistakes, unintentionally or with malice aforethought. If I have low tolerance for the way things are, if I think people and events in the world *should be a certain way*, I am going to have a long string of miserable days. I am going to have big-time stress, just about every day.

So there's a lot to give up. *Giving stuff up* is the access to creating a shift in who you are being. Am I being an angry, short-tempered, sharp-tongued person? Do I have a short fuse? Or am I being patient and considerate, aware of the possible worries and concerns of another? Am I gruff and bossy, aware only of my own busy and important schedule? Or am I polite and respectful of another, aware that his time concerns are as important to him as mine are to me? The difference between these two contrasting internal states can be observed in the effectiveness of your interactions: How smoothly and quickly do things get done? How satisfactory are the respective outcomes? Are things moving forward or are there obstructions and delays? Is your blood pressure rising (figuratively or literally) throughout the day or are you crossing items off your to-do list? In short, who you are being determines how you are doing. You get to choose, and the access to choosing is giving stuff up.

What might there be to give up? Self-importance, for starters. I have been very self-important, and this quality will easily pop to the surface. When I am being this way I am a boring know-it-all; people are left with, "what a stuck-up jerk". With an awareness of this tendency there is an ability to give it up, to choose to be another way. Without awareness, I'm just that jerky know-it-all. For example, for the last ten years I've been teaching postgraduate orthopedics to chiropractors. I teach various modules on the spine and the extremities, and I teach the course review. I've always been an effective instructor, and evaluations by the course participants indicated that their time was well spent. However, there were always one or two evaluations that were highly unfavorable, as if these people had been offended in some personal way. Their comments were often down-right derogatory. I could never understand this, thinking that I was always well prepared and covered the material effectively.

There was a missing ingredient to which I had failed to pay attention. The *personal* ingredient. I was unaware of, blind to, *who I was being.* My attitude was, "I'm the expert, I've got the answers, and I'm here to give them to you." Not much room in this for collegial conversation. Not much room for the students (who, after all, were practicing chiropractors) to share their experiences, to offer opinions different from those held by the instructor, who of course had been a star student in his day. Ouch. I can see in retrospect how an independent thinker would loathe such an instructor. If I was my own student, I would have been very unhappy. Most people were not offended, or were too kind to be offended because I was hard-working and diligent, but some people were very displeased. Fortunately, in the last few years I have been able to create a change, to cause a shift.

I chose to give up the position of knowing it all, the attitude of self-importance. Now, what I bring to these courses is, "I'm a colleague and I have some information to share. Yes, I'm an expert, *and* I'm interested in your contribution and what you have to bring to the discussion." When a question is posed, or when a statement I have made is challenged, I don't experience it as an attack but rather as an opportunity to dig deeper, to investigate whether something new can be uncovered. What a difference! I have more freedom; they have more freedom. Not only is some education getting done, but authentic human interactions are occurring as well. There is the possibility of some fun, some enjoyment, in the context of an intense academic experience. People are both learning and laughing. Of course, my old reactions lurk beneath the surface, but my *awareness* is the key to how things go.

Another consequence of my giving stuff up is an ability to generate an intention for my students. Generating intentions provides a purpose for your actions and interactions. Without an intention I'm adrift, rudderless, my purposes are unclear. Without an intention my actions are random, unfocused. Without an intention my results are haphazard, maybe even sloppy. For example, when I was in college the grades I produced varied wildly, ranging from "C" through "A". The courses I "liked" I did well in; in the ones I didn't like (there were a lot of those) I did poorly. Yes, it was the 1960s, but more to the point, I had no focus, no guiding principles, no discipline. I was self-indulgent, letting my likes and dislikes determine my outcomes. I had no *intention* for my time in college. When I began my chiropractic education, I had a clear purpose: I was going there because I actively *chose* to, rather than being pulled along by circumstances, and I was going to produce results in line with my ability. I intended to graduate first in my class. In fact, I graduated second, but what I learned along the way has served me throughout my career. I had brilliant instructors and a great education. I loved school; I intended it to be great and it was.

I might have learned something from that experience, but I didn't because it was fairly easy for me to be intentional about school. It's familiar for me to have success in that environment. What has more recently become clear is that success with *people* is critical to health, happiness, and well-being. Success with people comes from *being with* people: What are their interests and concerns? What's important to them? What's going on in their world? This is distinct from what's happening with me, what are my likes and dislikes, what am *I* feeling? If my concerns are focused on "What am I feeling?", then I'm going to miss out on everything that's going on over there with you, and our interaction is probably going to fail. I'm not present to you, I'm present to me. My familiar responses, reactions, and thought patterns are right there, readily available, and our interaction becomes mechanical, preprogrammed. There's no need for new thinking or creativity in a relationship if I've seen it before and know how it's going to go.

There are other possibilities. I am learning to create a shift in my attention, from me to you. When my focus is on you, the other person, something new becomes available. In my postgraduate teaching I am intentionally creating that shift. My concern is with them. What's going on over there? What do they have to say? What has occurred in their experience that relates to the topic being discussed? I invite their contribution and specifically say that. I *intend* the educational experience to be useful and valuable for them. Recently, I received a phone call from one of my students, a chiropractor from San Francisco who had taken my orthopedics review course and will shortly take the first part of his board exams. "I didn't know how to prepare for the exam," he said. "I didn't know what to study or how to study. I thought I'd take it, just to try it, and then maybe pass it on the second or third try." He continued, "Now I have a plan. I'm making the time to study, things are coming together, and I believe I have a chance to pass the board." He experienced this shift in intention and direction out of participating in my review class.

A few months ago I completed teaching two consecutive modules in one location. I taught that class one weekend a month for six months. This was unusual; typically I teach one module at a particular site and might come back twelve or eighteen months later. So this group had the full Lemberg experience. Really. At the end of the last session, most of them came over to express their personal thank-yous, and two said they had changed their practice styles as a result of having been in my classes for six months! This was a direct fulfillment of one of my intentions, that is, to have caused a shift in my students' methods of practice. And, this was particularly gratifying since one of my instructors had caused a similar shift in me in 1985, when I was his student in a postgraduate course. None of these results would have occurred had I not created intentions for my classes, and had I not been *listening keenly* for the interests and concerns of my students.

Likewise with my patients. I've been treating a guy named Tom, a financial analyst in his early fifties. Tom had lower back pain, radiating pain into his right thigh, and neck pain and stiffness. He hadn't been able to turn his head comfortably to the left for years. At our first meeting I asked Tom about his exercise program. He didn't have much of one, had been "pretty out of shape" for a long time. He used to run, but in the past his doctors had told him to stop, that running was "bad" for him. I asked him what type of exercise he would be interested in doing. He said, "I used to enjoy running. I'd like to do that but everybody says I can't." I said, "OK, let's see what the physical exam shows." Tom's examination demonstrated biomechanical losses consistent with his history, but there was nothing that would prohibit him from running. I said, "Tom, once your pain is reduced, would you like to start running?" He looked at me in frank amazement. "Do you think I can?" he asked. "Yes, I do," I replied. "There's nothing here that says you can't run. In fact, it will be good for you."

Within three weeks Tom was much better and within six weeks his pain had resolved. He started running, building up to thirty minutes or more three times a week, and regained most of the mobility in his neck. He lost six pounds, his facial pallor was replaced by a soft glow, and his eyes were brighter. He also reported that, on his own, he had significantly reduced his anti-anxiety medication. "I'm not so nervous now," he said. "I feel a whole lot better, in every way." What had occurred here? Well, treatment certainly helped, but the most important factor in the restoration of Tom's well-being was his running. He could run, and therefore he wasn't "sick". There wasn't "something wrong with him"; there was no permanent "damage".

My role? Well, in addition to my usual function of restoring more normal biomechanics and reducing pain, I had an intention for Tom in the area of fitness and well-being. My intention was that he run. Tom took this on and produced great results. In the absence of my specific intention, my only service would have been that of pain management. In that case, many opportunities would be missed. How are these opportunities identified?

Well, mostly by listening. Listening to the other person, his concerns and fears, his goals and aspirations. Listening for an opening in which that person can express himself. This kind of rigorous listening is possible when I am able to give stuff up, in particular, to give up listening to the racket going on in my own head. If I can do this then I can be *present* to the conversation I'm having with another, present to what's going on with him or her. What else is there to give up, in the moment? Plenty. For example, my opinions, prejudices, preconceptions, and attachments to how I want things to turn out. Now, letting go of this mental flotsam and jetsam is a learned skill and takes a lot of practice. You do not "master" this skill to the extent that you no longer have your own internal conversation. That's always there; what you learn is the ability to give it up in the moment and cause yourself to be present. You develop some skill in the area of *velocity*, some skill in giving stuff up quickly.

How does this relate to living a great life? Well, relationships are a large part of living, and in relationships there's always something to give up. Now, again, I'm not talking about *denial*. I'm not talking about denying yourself anything or denying your *feelings*. I am suggesting that living based on "feelings" is going to create a world of hurt. I dwell on my feelings, my feelings create moods, my actions are based on my moods ("I didn't feel like doing that"), and ultimately I create a mess. Another way might be: OK, I'm feeling that, he or she said or did this or that, this or that happened, now what do I intend to cause in this relationship or situation? I take responsibility, rather than being a victim.

And, since I'm responsible, why not have my world be great? Am I still sad, in my life? Yes, here and there. Do I still get upset? Yes, and a better formulation might be, do I still choose to be upset? Looked at from this perspective, being upset is a state I've chosen. So I can be upset, give up being upset, and choose to be something else. I don't mean to be simplistic here, or to gloss over the losses and tragedies in a person's life. It's a random universe. Stuff happens. It takes discipline and work, every day, to give up the upsets and create something new. Really, sometimes I just don't want to. I would rather wallow in whatever upset I have at the moment. Maybe it's a *big* upset. So I wallow, and I know I'm not going to wallow too long. There's too much great stuff going on, I'm choosing that it be great, and it's time to start taking action and producing some results.

How do I give up being upset? By taking responsibility. It's my world, after all. The other person didn't make me upset; I chose that. Yes, this or that happened. If I'm upset about it, that's my choice. Now, recognizing that, maybe I can choose something else. In this way I cause a shift from a victim state, from a reaction state, to one of being responsible. I get to say how my life is going to go, in the face of whatever circumstances. Every survivor of the Holocaust went through this process, in their daily struggle to create *living* in the face of particularly desperate circumstances. Several United States Presidents, including Abraham Lincoln, Ulysses S. Grant, and Bill Clinton, have reached the pinnacle of both service and power after a childhood of poverty. Persons with disabilities are faced with these choices every day, when the simple activities of daily living become daunting tasks requiring preparation and concentration. It is easy to forget, if our bodies are whole and our homes secure, how difficult life can really be. If my biggest concerns have to do with people, that is, my relationships, then I will undertake a course of self-study, learn about myself and learn about people, and begin to empower myself and my relationships.

How can I empower the people around me? First, by causing myself to have a great day, intentionally, regardless of what happens. And, stuff will happen. But, it's a great day. I'm alive, aren't I? (As my stepfather says, "Consider the alternatives".) Manage the circumstances, intend some useful outcomes, take the actions to get there, and keep going. Again, I'm not suggesting this is easy to do, or having succeeded today, it will be easy tomorrow. There are always new circumstances, new stresses. *Velocity* is the key. Be upset, worry, wallow a little, and then give it up with velocity. Practice does improve velocity. The result, being-in-the-moment or being present, is a kind of *centering*. The people in your environment will notice and may actually discover "centering" themselves.

Next, I can intentionally choose to have the people around me be great. This intention creates great interactions. Again, taxi drivers provide a concrete example. Everybody knows about New York cab drivers. They're rude, dangerous, and charge too much to unsuspecting out-of-towners.

And, of course, you can never get a cab when you need one. If that's my expectation, then that's probably what I'll get. Instead, I expect my cab drivers to be polite, knowledgeable, and safe. I intend to get a cab, and quickly (within reason, matching my intention with what's happening at the moment in the universe, such as it's raining and I'm in the theater district). Interestingly, most of the time my taxi intentions are fulfilled. Occasionally there's a clunker, but my experience is that these men and women are hardworking individuals, usually supporting spouses and children. They are mostly foreign nationals and their English is more than adequate (in contrast, I only have a smattering of words in other languages). And they are invariably polite. I am polite and courteous, recognizing them as service workers, and they are polite in return, recognizing me as a customer. I intend our interaction to be positive and useful, not adversarial and upsetting. In this state, I can have the experience of a cab driver as a skilled professional. It works.

I can intend for all the service people in my life to be great: my handyman, the guys in my garage, my doormen, checkout people at the supermarket, my delivery people, the counterman at my deli, my butcher, my magazine store guys, customer reps at my telephone company, salespeople in clothing stores, all of them. Mostly, they are great. These interactions start with my being great with the other person. I expect things to go well. I am respectful, friendly, and interested in them as people. Now, these encounters may not always be successful, but that doesn't mean I'm going to be upset—not for long, anyway, when I remember to give it up. What I am is human, and I can recognize that humanity in another. Of course, this is an ongoing project.

What about relationships with my family, friends, colleagues, and coworkers? It may be more challenging to have these relationships be great because of the shared history: things I did and said, things they did and said, the miscommunications, failed expectations, and disappointments that are part of most relationships. There's more to give up here. The relationship will not work out, I can't cause myself to be great in this relationship, if I'm not willing to give up my opinions, assessments, and judgments of what occurred in the past. This is not a matter of pretending. Nor is it a matter of being inauthentic, or of ignoring past hurts. It does take communication, straight talk, saying what there is to say about the past events I am still carrying around with me. This takes work, work on myself.

This is the thorny part. How to say what I need to say without making the other person the culprit and me the innocent victim. Again, what is my intention? If my intention is to assign blame, to present the "facts" so that I am right or I am justified, there won't be much room for resolution. The other person is still "wrong". On the other hand, I could say, "This is how I interpreted events. This is what I felt and how I reacted, and this is what I thought." Now, there's an opportunity for the other person to share his or her interpretation of those same events. There can be some clearing of the background, and an opportunity to create something else. Such a dialogue takes courage.

The bad news is that these conversations don't get any easier. Something occurred, you have something you want to say to a person, and the habitual tendency is to bottle it up, to "let it go". But when you're with that person the next time, the interaction is colored by the failed encounters of the past. They're affected by what you wanted to express and didn't, about how you experienced something the person did or said, how it occurred for you. If we could speak up in the moment, not blaming, not showing how the person was wrong, but rather describing *our* experience, things might go differently.

If I can do this quickly, as near to the moment of the interaction as possible, rather than ignoring my experience and ultimately being inauthentic, then the other person can communicate in turn, and neither of us will add anything extra to the "baggage" we carry around inside our heads. Our next encounter may be more intimate, more authentic, because we've experienced the other person's authenticity and courage, and we have expressed ourselves rather than withholding.

This method of communicating takes practice. It's challenging because it contrasts sharply with habits we have built up over a lifetime. The reward is relationships that assist, rather than hinder, growth; relationships that provide something rather than take something away; relationships that foster, rather than stifle, personal creativity; relationships that are satisfying, stimulating, and loving. That's a pretty big payoff. And, I have to put something in to get something out.

Now, what do I intend for myself and what do I intend for others? For myself, I intend to be healthy and happy. Being healthy relates to everything we're discussing here. Being happy relates to being self-expressed. Self-expression does not imply saying everything that pops into my head or doing something just because I *think* of doing it. Self-expressed does not mean *selfish*. Rather, I suggest the self-expressed person is naturally appropriate to his circumstances. He is aware of others in his environment and sensitive to their issues, needs, and concerns. Self-expression, that is, expression of the self, relates to creativity. This might involve bearing children and raising a family. It might involve creating and developing your own business or enterprise. It might involve new areas of study, such as a new language or art form. What are your areas of interest? What are the fields in which you might experience expression of your *self?*

One day, years ago, in acting class, I had just finished doing a scene with my acting partner, and my teacher, Greg, turns to me with a puzzled look in his eyes. He says, "David, when I talk to you I don't know which side of your brain is listening". Everybody got a good laugh out of that, including me. I was a successful chiropractor, fifteen or so years older than most of my acting classmates, most of whom worked nights at bars and restaurants. Greg's point was that I had been "acting", deliberately and methodically, rather than being spontaneously in the moment and expressing myself naturally. He went on to say, "there is no place for science in the arts", a statement which could be challenged in its superficial message, but it had great value for me, then and now. I saw that I could throw away the crutch of bringing the science "tool" to my artistic endeavors, even though the "science" means of expression was more familiar and safe. Particularly, in acting, it was the safety that needed to be jettisoned, and I think Greg was pointing to this.

I believe that many of us, or even most of us, are both scientists and artists, and we have deep, abiding interests in these two great topic areas. For the most part, though, we don't know it. It has been bred or, figuratively, beaten out of us. I propose that neglect of one area can bring malaise and dissatisfaction. A critical part of a person's expression is ignored, suppressed, or repressed. We don't know why we're unhappy, we just are. We don't know why we're so stressed out, we just are. We don't know why our jobs are so dull, they just are. Likewise, our relationships. Same old, same old. Day after day.

How can we cause a shift in this enervating routine? By intentionally looking for what's missing, and putting it in. I'll propose a few characteristics of human beings. A human being is naturally curious and inquisitive. A human being naturally likes to take things apart and put them back together. This is the science part. A human being naturally likes to make something out of nothing, to create something that is an expression of who he or she is, that is, a self-expression. This is the art part. What's missing, for many adults and probably many children, are expressions of these essential human qualities: curiosity/discovery, analysis/synthesis, and creativity/invention. A first step is to actually notice these activities or qualities are missing. Often, it's been so long, we've forgotten there's any possibility at all for creative pursuits. We've forgotten we used to like to do these kinds of things.

So, a person could say, "My life is dull and uninteresting. Get up, go to work, go home. Everything's routine. Nothing is new." The long-term results can be dissatisfaction, stress, and stress-related disorders and diseases such as insomnia, hypoglycemia, chronic fatigue syndrome, fibromyalgia, and irritable bowel syndrome. How to change? The first step in causing a shift is to answer the question, "Who's responsible?" Well, I am. Next, identify what's missing: expressions of the essential human qualities. The next step for me is to be intentional and put stuff that is missing back in my life. Things such as learning to play the piano. Or taking a photography class. Or going to a museum or a dance concert. Or going to graduate school. Or taking any of dozens of human development courses. Or volunteering.

For others, creative expression might manifest in repairing the roof, growing vegetables, building model planes, designing jewelry, or crocheting sweaters. You know, all the things you've been wanting to do and have put off doing because you say you don't have the time. Well, this stuff is just like exercise. Right now, you don't have the time. There is no time in my busy schedule for exercise. What there is to do is make the time. Reorganize my schedule. Be efficient. Sleep less. Some people accomplish a lot in their twenty-four daily hours, moving skillfully from project to project. You know the business management cliché, "If you need something done, find a busy person to do it." Being effective with our daily allotment of time is simply a matter of intentionality. Again, I don't mean to be simplistic. But that's all there is to it. And, like most areas we're discussing, this effectiveness is a developed skill.

Here's another possible conversation that maintains the steady state of dispiritedness and ennui. I might not be good enough or I might fail. Therefore I don't even begin a new activity. Here, the thought of not having enough time perfectly justifies the fear of beginning something new. And, yes, this fear can be so overwhelming that nothing new ever gets started. I can offer a few comments here. These internal conversations are automatic mechanisms, part of being a human machine. In other words, one human mechanism is to seek safety and shelter, and avoid new contacts or circumstances because they might be dangerous or fatal. However, a contrasting human mechanism is to explore and discover, to seek out new experiences that would increase one's security and position. So, it's really a matter of identifying the conversation that is in place and then having the possibility of choosing another. Also, it's empowering to acknowledge *what is present*. Yes, I have fear; now, *is the fear going to have me?* If the fear has me, not much is going to get done; I'm just going to be afraid. If I can shift to *I have the fear,* then there is the possibility of moving forward. OK, I'm afraid, or whatever, and I am going to do this and that anyway.

I am privileged to know many people for whom each day, pretty consistently, is a *great* day. Exactly how do they come to this place of creativity and enthusiasm? I suggest these qualities are self-generated, by choice. In other words, I can choose to be creative, engaged, and involved; enthusiasm will naturally flow from being these things. Or I can choose to be uninterested, bored, and unhappy, and just drift along. Again, the power comes from seeing that I have a choice. Do things go wrong in these persons' lives, sometimes horribly wrong? Yes. Do they pull themselves up off the deck and cause themselves to get back in the creative flow? Yes. It takes courage, determination, and love to keep going. Remember, the default condition for machines is entropy, that is, disorder or randomness. If a machine isn't maintained and serviced properly, it will break down. Likewise with human lives. So a great life, a happy, creative, and fulfilled life, requires causality and intentionality.

What about relationships? What would it be like to bring curiosity/discovery, analysis/synthesis, and creativity/invention to my family, friends, patients, and colleagues? What do I intend for the people in my life? Specifically, what do I intend for the *lives* of the people in my life? Well, I intend for people to be fully self-expressed. I intend for people to discover what they're good at and take that to the limit. I intend for people to dive into new areas and activities, if that's what they choose to do, and investigate and explore what they are capable of becoming.

Think about what a wonderful machine the human body is. Our built-in equipment includes state-of-the-art computers, audiovisual systems, environmental sensors, food processors, and self-contained transport. What's it all for? What purpose does this astoundingly complex mechanism serve? Well, I'm not certain of the "ultimate" purpose, but I suspect that a major purpose is one of *opportunity* and *possibility.* This remarkable machine is available to me so that I can do stuff. What kind of stuff? Well, basically, *create things*. Engage in experiences. Create new things, things that haven't been available before. Also, *provide things*. Provide things for family, friends, and community. If I can provide something, or create something, that's a contribution. Others might be stimulated to provide or create other things, and our experiences continue to expand and grow. The possibilities of life on earth (and, maybe soon, off earth) expand exponentially as people engage in the question, "What am I here for? Who am I here to be? What am I here to do?"

My brain is a massively parallel central processing unit; my five senses are penultimate data acquisition systems; my respiratory and digestive pathways are energy collectors, refiners, and distributors; and my bones, muscles, and ligaments provide easy transport for the entire structure. It's quite a machine, and I own one. So do you. Now, no one's telling me what to do with this priceless toy. I get to choose and, being human, as distinct from being perfect, some of my choices will be brilliant and others will be egregious mistakes. It's useful for me to continue to remember that life is a gift. There are specific functions I can perform and purposes I can fulfill. I can be aware of and alert to opportunities for performing and fulfilling these purposes and functions.

It's certainly easy to get stuck, to have long runs of "bad days", to keep thinking that things didn't work out the way they were supposed to, to continue to be attached to the pain of the past. Some people don't function this way, they just shake off the disappointments and move on. More typical is worrying and wallowing, dwelling in the errors and the mistakes. But in this more common behavior, we give up our ability to learn, adapt, and change. Growth is stunted because the focus is backward. One benefit here is that it's safe to look backward, that stuff has already happened. It may not be so nice, but it is known. What hasn't happened, what's not known, that could be the scary part, but that's where the growth is. That's where the newness is, that's where the fun is, that's where the human-ness is. So what is there to do? Acknowledge our inertial tendencies to look to the past, and to keep intentionally refocusing our thoughts, actions, and interactions toward the future. And to keep remembering that the future starts with the now.

Being human is a process of becoming. Each of us, moment to moment, occupies a particular fluid point, on our own personal continuum, in the growth-and-development dimensional space of our existence. This point of view can provide a lot of tolerance. And, as I give myself some room to be less than perfect, give myself some room to be *becoming,* I find I have more tolerance for the "imperfections" I experience in others. Being more comfortable with myself, I am better able to *be with people.* Being with people, of course, is the key to just about everything.

Another empowering perspective is that nothing is fixed, we're always transitional. That is, things are the way they are now *and* there are all these possibilities. This is not change for change's sake. This perspective doesn't excuse avoiding taking a stand and staking out territory, but rather allows one to be in the flow and acknowledge the universality of change. Being firmly rooted in the present *and* available to the possibility of change is a powerful combination.

Being fit and healthy supports all one's purposes. The time it takes to maintain optimal health is time well spent. One's efforts in the *being* realm support the physical realm, the physical supports what gets done in the world, and so on, reflexively throughout life. It's very possible to neglect one of these areas and still have a wonderful existence. I suggest that achievement in both realms provides a fulfilling and satisfying life, flowing from the active pursuit of excellence and expression.

Let's take a look now at actually *being well* in the physical realm. Our approach to fitness involves posture, stretching, weight-training, and running (as an example of aerobics). Then we'll present sound, sensible nutritional information that can be applied successfully by everyone. We'll discuss developing a powerful relationship, a relationship that works, with your sports physician. Finally, we'll investigate *coming back stronger,* a modern approach to recovery from injury.

CHAPTER 4

▼

VISUALIZATION: YOUR MIND
AS YOUR MIRROR

The notion of posture is a good place to start in any comprehensive discussion of fitness. But posture is a tricky subject. People have a lot of emotional baggage relating to the word itself. "Good posture" implies strength of character, discipline, definiteness of purpose, being in action, stick-to-it-iveness. "Bad posture" connotes low self-esteem, sloppiness, general failure. We take this particular issue rather personally.

Many of my patients spontaneously offer their own assessments, commenting "Oh, I have bad posture", during the inspection portion of a physical examination. I vividly remember the words of my fourth grade teacher, Mrs. Wiseman: "David, you look just like a pretzel". Sometimes I think I have spent the rest of my life compensating for her observation. Many people are uncomfortable with their bearing, thinking their stomachs bulge too much, their shoulders slump forward, or their buttocks stick out too far. Something's wrong, it shouldn't be this way, and we just don't measure up. When I was a boy, "good posture" meant chin up, stomach in, shoulders back. This was supposed to represent a military bearing; most importantly, one was admonished to "stand up straight". This imagery persists. Today, when I ask someone to show me "good posture" or to "stand up straight", he will invariably suck in his stomach, stick out his chest, and pull his shoulders back.

People with good posture do "stand up straight", but they do so with ease, rather than by maintaining any fixed position. Yes, the chin is up. Yes, the stomach is flat, but not because the person is "holding in" his stomach. And, no, the shoulders are not pulled back. The shoulders are resting comfortably on the rib cage, the head of the arm bone is in line with the outside of the hip, and both are in line with the ankle (Figure 4.1).

Good posture describes a biomechanically efficient, easy, aligned body position. Good, effective posture is definitely straight, neither slumped nor rigid. You could imagine the various sections of your body stacked one on top of the other, like building blocks: the head rests on the chest, which rests on the abdomen, which rests on the pelvis, which rests on the thighs, which rest on the calves, which finally rest on the feet. In fact, your body's weight is sequentially transmitted level by level into the floor, exactly like this. Now, really, when's the last time you thought about the efficient mechanical functioning of your body? Well, just like every other *system*, posture requires proper maintenance or it will begin to fail.

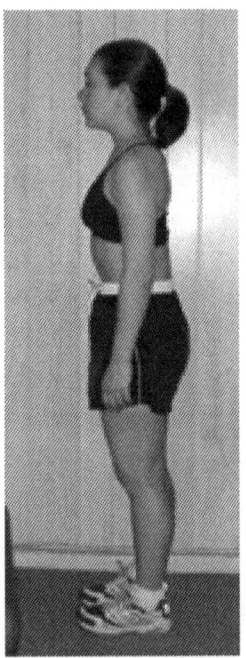

Figure 4.1

How do most of us spend most of our time? Probably in a seated position, whether in a chair at work or on the sofa or in a recliner at home. All this sitting has a weakening effect on the abdominal muscles; these structures begin to sag. Since we're very busy, we need both hands for work while we talk on the telephone. The phone is held between the arm and the shoulder, eventually causing significant strain to the neck and upper back. Men carry briefcases and attachés, working women may also carry heavy handbags in addition to their briefcases. Throughout the day there are opportunities for the development of inefficient, wasteful, muscle-tightening patterns. If the patterns are repeated frequently they become habits, creating postural distortions and cascading muscular tightness. Therefore, less-than-optimal posture is not merely a question of aesthetics. Postural inefficiencies may lead to various deeply rooted pain patterns in either the back, the extremities, or both locations.

Most of us would benefit from some attention to our posture. We'll look at several techniques for improving postural mechanics. Please consider that your posture represents the habits of a lifetime and change will come slowly. I suggest you approach these corrections as a process. I explain to my patients that for most of the day, they'll forget these recommendations, and simply keep reminding themselves to incorporate the corrections. Over time new, more efficient habits will develop. Also, many postural corrections involve imagery and are more of a *thinking* or a *seeing* rather than a *doing*. This *imaging* takes practice and you might not experience that anything is *happening*. Keep going. Remember that postural change occurs over weeks and months and is not a function of something you are *doing*. You are retraining muscular memory, establishing new patterns, new connections between your brain and your muscles. You are restoring an ease of movement, a natural grace that was present in childhood. It's a process.

Here's a wonderful mechanism for recapturing a long, vertical line of action, which runs from the tip of your head to your connection with the floor (your feet). I was introduced to this concept long ago by Finis, one of my ballet teachers. The image is called, "hitch your sternum to a star". The sternum is the breastbone, and you imagine a string attached to a star in the sky, extending all the way down to attach its other end to your sternum. Thus, you imagine a connection, a line, between your breastbone and a star. Dangle from that string like a puppet. The string holds you up in a true, vertical line. If your sternum is hitched to a star, you are always upright. There is no slumping, no collapsing of the chest. The chest is naturally broad and wide without being puffed out or thrust forward. It is simply lifted, elevated by its vertical connection with the heavens.

There are several things that "hitching your sternum to a star" is not. It's not "pull the shoulders back and stick out the chest". It's not "lift the chin up and stick out the neck". It's not "lift up both shoulders". It's not "stop breathing". I have witnessed all these errors during attempts to reproduce "hitching your sternum to a star". If you can see the image clearly, see the string linking a bright star and your chest, there will be a natural elevation, a very subtle lifting, of your sternum. You will be standing straight, erect and upright. Dangle from that string like a marionette. And, breathe while you're doing this. There will be a tendency to stop breathing and to begin *holding* the new position. Resist this tendency. Find the image and intentionally breathe. Train yourself to attain the new posture and be breathing at the same time. Also, give yourself room to fail. Practice definitely "makes perfect".

Here's another technique for improving posture and presentation. Most posture gurus, starting with our grandmothers, told us to suck in our stomachs. Mr. Moscowitz, my gym teacher in high school, told us quite frankly to "suck in that gut"! Some dance teachers offered no better instruction. "Hold in your stomach" was a common correction. Also, "tuck your pelvis under". This particularly insidious "correction" would lead to the development of large rear ends, since "tucking under" is initiated by contracting the gluteal muscles. You could often guess correctly where someone new in class had been studying by gauging the size of their posteriors. Big behinds meant they were from the "tucking under" school.

Well, how do you flatten your abdomen and decrease the sway (lordosis) in your lower back? Again, we'll use an image to achieve effective posture. Imagine a rectangular plane, about eighteen inches wide and nine inches high, directly in front of your lower abdomen. Now, imagine another identical plane placed directly behind your lower back and upper buttocks. The image is to bring these two planes together, maintaining their vertical orientation, deep inside your body. This is a *seeing,* rather than a *doing.* As the two planes are brought together in your mental image, the physical result will be flattening of the stomach and lengthening of the muscles of the lower back. The abdomen will naturally be drawn in and up; the pelvis will naturally drop under, somewhat flattening the lumbar lordosis. The results are *not* created by intentional muscular action. You are neither sucking in the stomach nor tucking the pelvis under. The muscular action flows from your mental image; the clearer the mental image, the more precise will be the muscular effect. Maintain a natural breathing pattern as you are imaging the two planes coming together. The goal is to achieve postural balance and breathe at the same time.

Both postural images are challenging to initiate. You have no experience in doing them, nor, probably, much experience in using mental images to create physical action. You have experience in maintaining the habits of a lifetime; by their nature, habits tend to persist. They are habits. Be kind to yourself. No one *really* wants to change. The process of changing postural habits takes time. As I mentioned earlier, mostly you'll forget. Keep going, keep working on it, and there will come a time when the new pattern is established, when the new pattern is natural, when the new pattern is part of your being.

The development of any physical skill is a process. You keep working on it and one day it's there. For example, I remember the day, the precise dance class, when I learned to fit the choreographed steps to the music. I had started taking beginners' dance class in college, and soon thereafter moved to Amsterdam, in Holland. At that time, in the Amsterdam dance world there were no beginners classes for young adults. There were only a few teachers, and the classes they held were for the small community of professional dancers. So I took the classes that were available, the advanced classes. For the most part these classes were conducted in Dutch. The dancers and teachers knew some English, some of them had a good command of English, but they were Dutch and naturally the classes were given in Dutch.

Looking back on those days, taking those classes might have been the stupidest and the bravest thing I have ever done. I was clueless, literally almost starting from scratch, way behind in a class given in a language I couldn't understand. Fortunately, my teachers were kind and my class-mates, when they weren't laughing too hard, were helpful.

What a difficult and challenging process! Slowly, I began to be able to follow a choreographic sequence, began to string several phrases together with some degree of accuracy. After months of classes I could learn sequences involving sixty-four counts or so. Still, there's a difference between reproducing a sequence of steps and *dancing* the steps musically, that is, in time with the music—in other words, dancing on the beat, dancing a particular step or sequence of steps exactly in time with a particular musical note or phrase. I couldn't do that. I wasn't even close. Then one day Lynn and Fred came to town, two great jazz dance teachers from New York. The Amsterdam dancers had been talking about Lynn's arrival for weeks. She was a big topic of conversation: what had happened in her classes in previous summers, how great she was, how hard her classes were, and so on. Fred was a bonus: it was his first time teaching in Europe. If you were a dancer, Amsterdam was the place to be in Europe that summer. Lynn and Fred were both skilled and inspired teachers. They saw beyond my awkwardness and unrefined technique and related to me as if I, too, were a professional. Of course, when we met I was, at best, an advanced beginner.

There was wonderful anticipation about going to class: what type of music would be used, what new steps would be learned, what familiar, friendly steps would be reviewed, who would be there, would there be any new people in class that day. My technique improved over the next few weeks, but I still wasn't dancing to the music, not exactly. I would finish early, finish late, do the accented step on the wrong note, jumble the musical transitions. Then one fine day, one beautiful, sunny, summer day, it happened. It was toward the end of one of Fred's classes. The combination was syncopated, funky, and sexy. The men were dancing, six or seven of us, moving with fierce passion. And then the combination was done, the music over. I finished dancing exactly on the last note, and I noticed Fred staring at me, his jaw slightly open, eyes popping. "Great, David," he said. "Right on time." I had *never* been "on time" before. Miraculously, as it appeared to me at the time, I had learned to dance to the music. On that day I became a musical dancer, a skill that has lasted a lifetime. Developing a facility with these new postural images is exactly like becoming a musical dancer. You keep training, keep working on the skills, and then they become yours.

Let's look at the third imaging technique for attaining postural excellence. So far we've elevated and opened the rib cage and achieved an inner lift of the abdominal musculature. Now we'll address the position of the shoulder girdles. The shoulder girdle includes the humerus (arm bone), the scapula (the shoulder blade), and the clavicle (the collarbone). These three bones form the roughly semicircular shoulder girdle which is designed to rest on top of the rib cage. The connection between the shoulder girdle and rib cage is almost exclusively soft tissue. The only bony connection between these three bones and the rest of the body is a small coin-shaped joint between the collarbone and sternum. The shoulder girdle's attachment to the rib cage is essentially muscular. The nature of this attachment provides great mobility and flexibility: the arm can rotate through a 360-degree arc in both front-to-back and side-to-side directions.

There is a postural downside to this extensively muscular connection. Much opportunity exists for development of postural holding patterns, that is, inappropriate muscular contractions maintained for lengthy periods of time. We tend to interfere with the natural resting position of the shoulder girdle. Rather than letting our shoulders simply rest on their bony rib supports, we tend to hold them up. Most people's shoulders are in a continual state of mild elevation. This ongoing elevation is maintained by muscular contraction of a relatively broad, triangular sheet of muscle called the trapezius. Muscles are designed to contract and relax, so any persistent contraction of a muscle will have harmful consequences. Anaerobic muscular work produces lactic acid as a metabolic end-product. Normally these end-products are cleared by the local capillary circulation. However, persistent muscular contraction constricts local blood supply and lactic acid accumulates rather than being removed. The lactic acid build-up irritates local nerve endings, causing pain. The pain provokes further muscular contraction in an attempt to limit movement of the area (this is an involuntary response, a preconscious attempt to avoid additional pain).

Thus, a positive feedback loop is established, in which chronic muscular contraction produces pain which produces further muscular contraction. Eventually structures known as trigger points develop: these are local muscular nodules which can cause both local and radiating pain. Trigger points can be very uncomfortable. When a person says, "I have a painful knot in my shoulder", he's referring to a trigger point.

The typical origin of this painful cycle is inefficient posture, specifically relating to the shoulder girdles. For most of us, the position of these structures is not neutral but elevated, to a greater or lesser extent. The correction lies in letting go of the inappropriate muscular holding pattern, allowing the shoulder girdle to descend to its natural resting position. An image will assist in this process. Decades ago young farm workers carried milk jugs from the cowshed to the kitchen. These jugs, filled with milk, were suspended from a yoke which straddled the child's shoulders. The jugs hung straight down from the yoke, perpendicular to the ground. The yoke rested on the shoulders. There was no effort to hold the yoke up, no attempt to lift the yoke while moving. The weight of the milk in the jugs was distributed across the length of the yoke. The weight was distributed across the upper back of the child, and then passed sequentially, by involuntary gravitational forces, into the ground.

Imagine your shoulder girdles as this yoke; they rest gravitationally on your upper ribs. There is no holding, no upward tension in the surrounding musculature. Your shoulders float freely, lightly resting on your upper ribs, the weight of your arms hanging down into the ground. This image of your shoulders as a yoke will ultimately relax and lengthen the associated muscles. Those painful knots or trigger points will become less troublesome. Observe the position of your shoulders during the course of the day, particularly when you are sitting at your desk. Are your shoulders elevated? If so, don't pull them down. Simply let go, allowing the shoulders to return to their resting position on the upper rib cage. Don't pull them down; simply don't hold them up.

There are a few other structural considerations for producing effective posture. Stand so your weight is placed over the balls of your feet. You may feel very strange at first, as if you're falling forward, and you may think, "This can't be right". This was my own experience as a beginning ballet student. My ballet teacher, Don, would come over to me and shift my whole weight forward, bringing my weight over my metatarsal heads (the balls of my feet). I always felt as if I were going to keel over, and as soon as he moved away I would shift my weight back over my heels. Postural habits! Eventually I learned to trust this weight-forward position and began to distinguish when my weight was drifting back toward my heels.

All bodily action flows from this weight-forward position. You are "prepared" if your weight is forward. If your weight is back, back on your heels, in order to do anything you first have to shift your weight forward. For example, in boxing, a time-critical activity, you might be KO'd in the instant you are attempting to redistribute your weight. "He's back on his heels" is a common phrase used by boxing announcers to describe the fighter who is losing the match. Dancers must have their weight forward over the balls of their feet; beginning dancers are trained in this, as Don was training me.

Jumping involves lifting off from the metatarsal heads, not the heels. Similarly, when you land from a jump, the sequence is "toe, ball, heel". Weight is redistributed into the ground by landing toe first, then placing the ball of the foot on the floor, and lastly the heel lands. Dancers who haven't yet mastered this technique land with a pronounced thud. Skilled dancers not only can jump high, but land almost without a sound. You can identify the well-trained dancers simply by listening. And, of course, runners run from the balls of the feet: we push off from our metatarsal heads.

So bring your weight forward! This efficient posture prepares you for action without wasting activity. You are already prepared by having your weight forward. This postural correction in itself may help alleviate various foot-related aches and pains caused by chronic inappropriate distribution of weight. Also, since the body is a *system*, mechanical trouble of the foot and ankle may initiate knee, hip, and back disorders. The system functions as a unit.

The next image helps align the entire lower extremity. We all know people who "walk like a duck" or are "pigeon-toed". These rather unflattering descriptions refer to a failure of alignment of a person's thigh, leg, and foot. There are a variety of orthopedic conditions that cause alignment anomalies and require bracing or corrective surgery in childhood. I'm referring to postural inefficiencies that develop over time and become habits. The alignment distortion is corrected by an image: imagine a line down the front of your leg, connecting your hip joint, patella (kneecap), and first or second toe. The hip joints are located about eight or nine inches apart, on either side of the groin. This imagined line travels downward from the hip joint, crosses the middle of the patella, and extends down the calf to end between the first and second toes. This is a straight line, perpendicular to the floor and bent at the knee, which can be imaged whenever you're walking, running, riding a bicycle, or even swimming.

Some people turn their feet out when they walk; others turn their feet in. Many people's knees form the apex of an obtuse angle between their hips and ankles (resulting in what is termed an "increased Q angle"; often associated with generalized knee pain). The image of hip/knee/first–second toe alignment addresses these several inefficiencies at once. Again, it is a *thinking* rather than a *doing*. "Doing" something here will create more distortion; these postural imbalances can't be corrected by any conscious decision to use or not use one particular muscle. "Trying to fix it" may even cause pain in your hip, knee, or ankle. Visualizing a straight leg, with the muscular energy flowing down the leg from hip to knee to foot, will create effective muscular action. Coordinated movement associated with improved joint alignment will be the result.

When I began studying ballet, about a year after taking my first jazz dance class, I developed severe pain in both knees. At times the pain was burning; at other times it was an icy pain, traveling through the knee joints. This was not only painful, but scary. I loved my dance classes but there was a heavy price to pay for being there. I could take a lot of pain, but this was a *lot* of pain. Eventually I had the pain in every class, whether ballet, jazz, or modern dance. Fortunately, Don, my ballet teacher, was a master at teaching young adults and retraining their bodies to withstand the rigors and demands of ballet. What I needed to learn, basically, was correct knee alignment. Throughout the next many months, I learned I was inadvertently creating twisting forces at my knee joint. I was sending energy (creating muscular lines of force) down my thigh in one direction and down my calf in a different direction. These vectors of muscular action were not parallel, were not aligned, and crossed at my knee, resulting in a physiologic twisting or torsion of the soft tissues of the knee—the ligaments and knee cartilages. The twisting caused the burning, icy pain.

When I would bend my knees in a plié, whether in a parallel (toes facing forward) or turned-out position, my knees would be positioned over a spot somewhere to the inside of my big toe. Of course, this nonparallel, twisted-knee position was also my preparation for jumps. So everything I was doing in dance class was creating twisting forces in my knees. Don identified the problem and taught me to "realign the energy". He talked about "straight lines of energy" and "seeing the leg straight". In particular, he asked me to visualize a point about one-half inch below the middle of my knee, on the inside of my shin, and a point about one-half inch above the middle of my knee, on the inside of my thigh. In a turned-out demi-plié (knees bent half-way) he would ask me to rotate those two points outward so my knee would be aligned over my big toe. Remarkably, the more I was able to do this, the less pain I had. When I would forget, reverting to my habitual knee posture, the pain would return. After a year or so my knee pain completely resolved. I had straight, long legs and could dance pain-free.

A severe pain pattern was corrected basically by imagery. There was no talk of "tucking under" or "tighten this muscle" or "squeeze these muscles together". Alignment was paramount, and *thinking* the alignment, creating a mental image of the bony/muscular pattern, was *most* paramount.

The "straight energies" concept provides a powerful method for correcting postural distortions. It implies muscle length, not muscle shortening. Inappropriate muscular contractions, over time, create pain, either from the development of trigger points or the twisting lines of force that distort ligaments and joint cartilage. Muscle work is most efficient when muscles are imaged as "long". (By the way, you don't have to be tall to have long muscles. It is the relative length of one's muscles that we're considering; any given muscle can be shortened or lengthened.) In ballet, typical commands are "reach the energy through your toes" or "reach through your fingers". This "energy lengthening" creates a long, liquid line, graceful, strong, and light. "Long" muscles distribute forces and are more efficient along the length of the muscle, all the way from the origin to the insertion. Mental commands such as tightening, gripping, or contracting focus work in a narrow region of the muscle, the midpoint of its length, resulting in short, bunchy musculature. The physical manifestation of muscular work is directly related to how you *think* about what you are doing.

Muscle holding patterns create postural distortion and, eventually, pain. Posture-related pain can occur in most locations: in the neck; middle back; lower-back; shoulder; hip, knee, and ankle; and elbow and wrist. This pain can also cause headaches. Wouldn't it be great to eliminate this unnecessary pain? Pain is a consequence *and* there are consequences of pain. Pain typically causes local muscle contraction as a protective response. Energy is wasted in these muscle contractions, and if the muscular activity is a response to a postural mechanism, the process is perpetuated and the energy drain is ongoing. Energy derived from food, air, and water, intended to fuel normal body functions including brain activity and immune responses, is wasted in these prolonged muscle contractions. The person becomes fatigued and irritable, more susceptible to infection, more susceptible to digestive disorders, and even unhappy or depressed. Consider disorders such as chronic fatigue syndrome and fibromyalgia. These debilitated states are characterized by generalized fatigue, pain, weakness, and irritability. There are no current medical solutions for these syndromes. What if biomechanical corrections were part of the solution, part of the restoration of vibrant good health? I am suggesting exactly that. Eliminating unnecessary sources of physical pain might be an excellent beginning.

Let's look at a few more innocuous postural inefficiencies that might lead to malaise and discomfort. Often, when I ask a person sitting on my examination table to sit up straight, he will arch his lower back and stick out his chest. We discussed sticking out your chest earlier; now let's consider what's happening in the lower back. Arching or hyperextending the lower back shortens the local muscles. The arched position is part of normal mechanics, of course, but it's not a posture to be maintained more than briefly. If most people respond to the request to "sit straight" by arching the lower back, then it's reasonable to conclude they assume this arched position whenever they think of "standing straight". Such a person would develop lower back pain, at the very least.

I'll show my new patient how to sit straight (sitting so the lower back is neither rounded nor arched; a plumb line could extend vertically from the middle of the shoulder blades to the base of the spine). Then I'll say, "you probably feel as if you are slumped". The person agrees, and I'll explain, "You're now sitting straight. You feel slumped because you're used to sitting with an arched back". This is like the correction for shifting the weight over the balls of the feet. Initially you feel off-center because the inefficient "center" you have created and lived with for years is actually off-line.

Here's another one. When you're standing, how much of the time is your weight shifted onto one leg? Now, this is not a horrible crime. However, it would be useful to vary your standing position, shifting the weight onto the opposite leg, or even better, standing so your weight is evenly distributed on two legs (of course, with your weight forward over the balls of your feet!). Being aware of options, of the benefits of avoiding a habitual, inefficient posture, is the value here. Our goals are grace, balance, harmonious muscular action, and efficient utilization of our raw materials and natural resources.

Let's review. Good posture can be attained by everyone. It results not from muscular action per se, but rather from visual imagery. It is a *seeing* or *thinking*, rather than a *doing*. Here are the three key body images:

1. Hitch your sternum to a star.
2. Visualize a rectangular plane in front of your lower abdomen and another behind your lower back, and bring these two planes together, deep inside your body.
3. Visualize your shoulder girdles as a yoke and let them rest on top of your rib cage, allowing your shoulders to hang into the floor.

Other mechanical corrections include the following:

1. Standing with your weight over the balls of your feet.
2. Imaging straight-line energy from your hip to your knee to your big toe.
3. Increasing the time your weight is balanced on two feet, rather than having most of your weight shifted onto one leg.
4. When sitting, sit comfortably straight, so your back is neither arched nor slumped.

Whew! This is a lot. You might be thinking, "How am I ever going to remember all of this?" You'd be right. If I were in dance class and my teacher gave me seven major corrections I might retain a glimmer of one or two. Here's a suggestion: select one or two at a time and work on them. Make them your own; get comfortable with the imagery and the machinery. You'll feel different; you'll feel unbalanced. In fact, you'll be unbalanced for a while: you're redesigning your biomechanics, away from the "center" you've created, toward a center that actually balances your physical structure and creates a platform for efficient action.

What is this *center?* It is the balance point of the various weights that make up your body: your head, torso, arms, pelvis, and legs. For practical purposes, your *center* is located midway between the pubic bone and the umbilicus (bellybutton) and about two inches deep (midway between front and back). You locate and activate your center by using the body image for the lower abdomen (bringing the two rectangular planes together). An unbalanced "center" is produced by inefficient postures, which cause unequal muscular action and ineffective weight distribution. Balance those weights!

Keep going. Your postural habits are the habits of a lifetime, and I'm asking you to start creating new habits. You'll forget to use the new concepts, simply because the old habits are *habits.* That's OK. Keep remembering and the new mechanisms will become new habits. Painful trigger points will reduce and dissolve as long-term muscle contractions are released and capillary circulation is restored. More energy is available since it's not being wasted in *holding* your various pieces together. You might even discover that sleep is more restful. My grandmother was right when she pinched my cheek and commanded me to "stand up straight"!

CHAPTER 5

▼

HOW I LEARNED TO STOP WORRYING AND LOVE TO STRETCH

Stretching is a crucial component of maintaining physical well-being. Stretching prepares the body for work or exercise; it may be done after exercise as part of a cool-down, but for most of us, stretching needs to be done before activity. Lately there has been some commentary in various media that stretching is appropriate only after exercise, that the body is not warmed up sufficiently for stretching to be useful before exercise. In fact, stretching *begins* the warm-up process. Stretching has been poorly understood by most people who are not professional or competitive athletes, and ineffectively applied by many. I'll propose some useful guidelines so that stretching can produce the desired result.

What usually comes to mind when we think about stretching? "I don't have time." "It's boring." "Why do I have to stretch?" "I don't know how to stretch." "My muscles are too tight to stretch." "I remember once when I hurt myself stretching." With all this and more in the background, many people just won't begin their workouts by stretching. And we need to stretch. We do. Some people are so remarkably limber they can ignore the stretching mandate. But there aren't too many of these. I'm not one of them. You're probably not, either.

One of the first questions I'll ask a person who has experienced some sports-related strain or sprain is, "Did you stretch?" Invariably the answer is "No, I don't usually stretch. Should I? Could that have something to do with my injury?" Generally, yes, it does have something to do with your injury. Of course, stretching is not a panacea; even if you stretch beforehand you may incur a strain/sprain. Stretching as a practice, done consistently, goes far toward preventing avoidable injuries. Basically, if you haven't stretched, you haven't prepared properly for physical effort.

I remember going to my first dance class, entering the studio, my eyes wide with both anxiety and excitement, standing a little apart from every-body else. I wasn't quite sure if I wanted to be there, ready to turn around and walk out the door if the newness of it became too threatening. I recall watching the dancers' preparations: bending over, stretching the lower back and hamstrings; legs on the *barre,* stretching inner thigh muscles; side bends; neck rolls. Everything was being done to loosen up, lengthen the muscle groups, and get the blood flowing to the various body parts. I mimicked some of their actions for a few minutes and then the class started. Interestingly, much of the exercise in any dance class can be con-sidered *stretching.* Over the years I learned a lot of exercises designed for stretching. I learned that dance class is designed to lengthen muscle groups: to make short muscles long and lengthen your line. This is done by repetitive exercises that involve lengthening—stretching. So, stretching is a way of life for dancers, and dancers may be considered pretty well-rounded athletes. Later, I brought my dance training to every other sport and exercise program in which I participated. I incorporate everything I learned as a dancer and dance teacher into my treatment of patients.

Muscle length is the key concept here. As the muscle lengthens, it can contract with greater facility and be more efficient. Longer muscles can bear heavier loads and do more work. In dancer's terminology, a muscle that hasn't been stretched is "cold"; it needs to be warmed up before any useful, vigorous work can be done. Otherwise that muscle could be injured. Dancers stretch, and they stretch before doing anything else.

How to stretch? One of my office handouts describes stretches for the hamstrings, calves, and quadriceps (the large muscle group on the front of the thigh; the "quads"). This stretching routine is particularly useful for patients with lower back discomfort. The majority of my patients are business people and, of course, they're New Yorkers. They are success-oriented, goal-oriented people who don't have time for disabling pain (who does?). They want to get better *now* or sooner, and often attack the stretches, thinking they're really going for it. Of course, such an approach will cause further problems. I caught on to this behavior early and learned to suggest that stretching is a process, a slow one at that. You're not trying to get anywhere when you stretch, you're not trying to accomplish *something*. You're just stretching. It's pretty Zen.

Some things do change. In the old days, we used to do some stretches ballistically, by bouncing. You would bend over and bounce back up. Or you would sit on the floor with your legs extended in front of you, reach your torso forward, touch your feet with your fingers or hold onto your feet with your hands, and bounce and recover, bounce and recover, stretching your hamstrings and lower back. Lately, it's been shown that ballistic-type stretching is not physiologically effective, and may even lead to a higher percentage of injury. Slow stretching is the way to go.

Visualization is an important component of stretching. *See* the muscle in your mind; conceptualize it. Hold a visual image in your mind of the muscle group, where it comes from, and where it goes. Visualization helps establish a brain-muscle connection, training the muscle group by honing the neurologic relationships. Balance in dance or gymnastics is very much like this. Visualization is also useful in weight-training—you see the muscle in your mind as you perform the exercise. As a dancer, before every performance I would stand in the wings and visualize the choreography, the sequence of steps I would be dancing. While I was learning a dance I would follow the same process, rehearsing the steps in my mind throughout the day while doing other tasks. Of course I remembered to look both ways before crossing the street!

Athletes in other sports also utilize visualization. High jumpers visualize the technical elements of the run to the bar and see themselves rising into the air, floating over the bar, and dropping onto the cushioning. Figure skaters mentally practice their routines in the weeks and days leading up to a competition. Baseball players mentally rehearse and evaluate their batting stroke; basketball players visualize the mechanics of foul shooting. By methods that aren't easily measured or evaluated, visualization techniques improve physical performance. Visualization is also beneficial in the broad arena of human potential. The same simple methods can be applied to stretching and posture.

When you stretch, visualize the length of the muscle, including its origin and insertion, and see the muscle lengthening. Part of this lengthening may include reaching (extending energy) through the heel, or reaching through the heel down into the floor, or reaching through the tips of the fingers or tips of the toes. "Reach through your fingers", "reach through your toes", or "lengthen your arm" are commands heard in the dance studio. Another identical command is "reach the energy down through your toes", the result of which would be a straight knee and a long line. We admire the results of long lines and flowing energy in a professional dancer, competitive figure skater, or gymnast. This extension of line is the basis of effective stretching.

Don, my ballet teacher, employed a particular method to have us achieve longer legs. We would do an exercise standing at the *barre* in which one foot was pointed straight ahead. The exercise would last for four bars of music of eight beats each, that is, thirty-two counts. On each count we would tap the pointed foot on the floor, lengthening the leg on each beat. Don would say, "lengthen the leg one thirty-second of an inch on each count", so by the end of the exercise everyone's leg would be an inch longer. That's exactly what happened! When the music stopped, my big toe would be at least an inch further away on the floor than when I started. My leg didn't actually get longer anatomically, but rather the muscles had lengthened and the knee was fully extended. This is the approach to employ when stretching.

Let's start with hamstring stretches, basic to every stretching program. The hamstrings are a group of three muscles which originate on the ischial tuberosity, the rounded, bony protuberance you can feel under your buttock when sitting. The hamstrings comprise the muscle bulk of the back of the thigh, and insert on the upper part of the tibia (the shin bone). Tight hamstrings affect the mechanics of walking, running, and jumping. Tight hamstrings may lead to lower back pain, even if the back is otherwise normal, and may also result in knee pain and ankle pain. Therefore, most people would benefit from regular and consistent stretching of their hamstring muscles.

The hamstrings can be stretched in at least three different ways:

1. Bending over and touching your fingers to the floor.
2. Placing one leg up on a support with that leg at a slightly less than 90-degree angle to the standing leg.
3. Sitting on the floor with your legs straight out in front of you, holding onto your calves or ankles, and bending over your legs.

Any of these are good methods, but there is the possibility of straining a muscle if you are somewhat tight to begin with. The safest way to stretch your hamstrings is as follows. Lie on your back on an exercise mat (these are easily obtainable in any sporting goods store). We'll start by stretching the left hamstring group, so bend your right knee to form a 90-degree angle and keep the right foot on the floor (Figure 5.1). Draw the left knee toward your chest to release the hip joint, and then straighten that leg in the air (Figure 5.2).

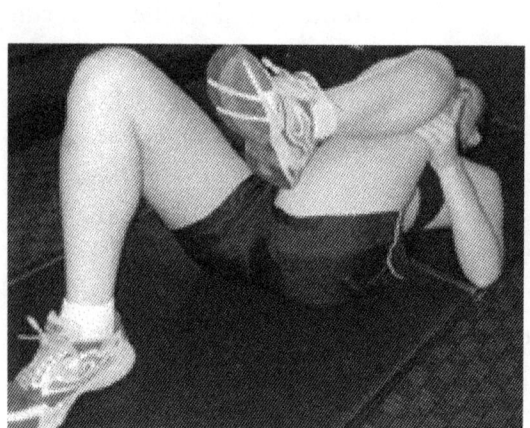
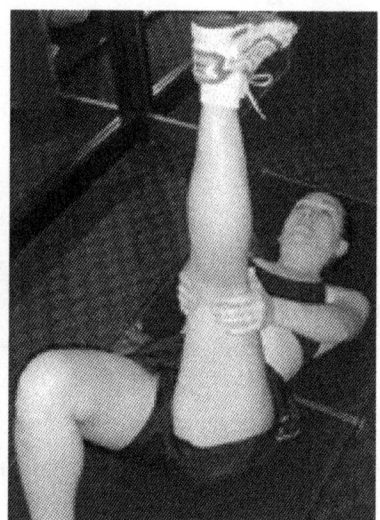

Figure 5. 1   **Figure 5. 2**

This will lengthen the hamstrings. You can maintain that leg in the extended position for a few seconds, possibly holding onto the calf and bringing the leg slightly and gently toward your head (increasing the flexed angle in the hip). Then bend the left knee, bring the knee toward your chest, and repeat.

I work on one leg for several minutes, possibly as long as five minutes. The goal is to be able to easily extend the knee so the leg makes a 90-degree angle with the floor. For many, this amount of flexibility may not be achieved for some time. Flexibility will increase over a number of weeks and months. It doesn't matter where you are when you begin. It doesn't even matter where you are when you finish. There is no better stretchability than this or that, no comparison between persons. No competition needs to exist concerning stretching. You are where you are. Any stretching is beneficial, and your flexibility *will* increase.

After completing this basic hamstring stretch, sit up and extend your legs in front of you. Gently round your torso over your legs, placing your hands on your knees, calves, or (if your hamstrings are very stretched) your feet (Figure 5.3). Breathe into your lower back, and stretch your torso down toward your legs as you exhale. Do this several times, feeling a gentle stretch in your lower back and hamstrings. Then, making sure to use your abdominal muscles for support, sit up and bring your right leg into a sign-of-four position. The other leg remains extended (Figure 5.4). Gently round your torso over your left leg, and repeat the breathing and stretching sequence several times. Then reverse your leg positions and repeat.

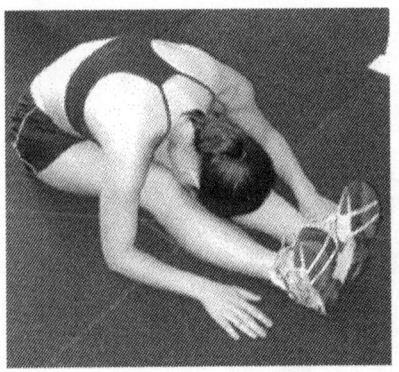 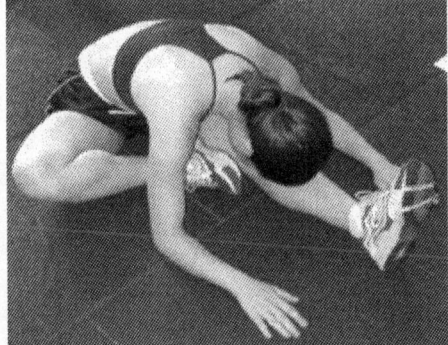

Figure 5.3   **Figure 5.4**

The next stretch in this three-stretch sequence involves the calf muscles, that is, the gastrocnemius and soleus muscles. The gastrocnemius is closer to the surface. The soleus lies beneath the gastrocnemius, closer to the tibia. The calf muscles point the foot and enable one to rise up on the balls of the feet. They are involved in jumping and all activities related to jumping. The calf stretch is the well-known "runner's stretch". You stand about twelve inches away from a wall and place both hands on the wall, at about shoulder height. Let's start by stretching the left calf. You stand on the right leg, with that knee bent at about 90 degrees. The right foot is facing forward, neither turned in nor turned out. The left leg is extended straight behind you, with the knee straight and the foot also facing forward, neither turned in nor turned out (Figure 5.5). How far behind you is the left foot? Far enough so that when you reach the left heel down to the floor, you feel a slight tug in the left calf. The stretch involves reaching the left heel into the floor (the left heel is touching the floor), and maintaining that line for about fifteen or twenty seconds. Then switch legs, stretching the right calf, and repeat both sides. Key aspects of the calf stretch are to keep both feet facing forward and have your weight placed over the front, bent leg. The deep calf muscle, the soleus, may be stretched in isolation as follows: Set up for a typical left calf stretch, with the left leg straight behind you. Lower the left heel to the floor and feel the stretch in the left calf. Now bend the left leg. The bent-knee position will stretch the soleus.

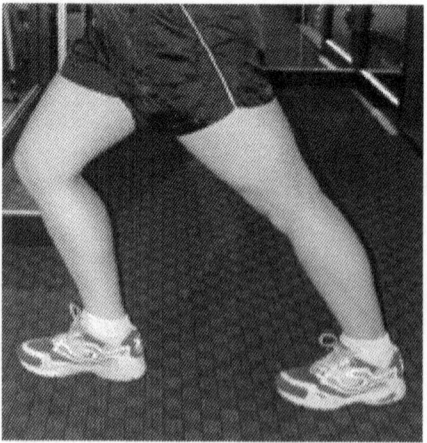

Figure 5. 5

The third stretch in this sequence works the quadriceps, the large muscle group on the front of the thigh. The quadriceps extends the leg at the knee; part of it (the rectus femoris) flexes the thigh on the hip. Let's start by stretching the left quadriceps. Stand on the right leg near a wall and lightly place your right hand on the wall for balance. Bend your right leg slightly, bend over, and grasp the left ankle in your left hand; then return to an upright position with the standing leg (right leg) straight and the working leg (left leg) bent at the knee, with your left hand holding the left ankle and placed behind the left buttock (Figure 5.6).

Your left knee should be near your right leg, so that the left leg is parallel to the rest of your body rather than turned out. Now, reach the left thigh down into the floor, so that the left thigh eventually becomes aligned with the right thigh (Figure 5.7). You will experience a stretch in the quadriceps running from the hip to the knee, and as a result the left heel will come closer to or even touch your left buttock. Don't bend at the hips and tilt forward. Don't pull the left heel to the buttock. The stretch occurs as a result of reaching down the left thigh. This creates a long line and a longer

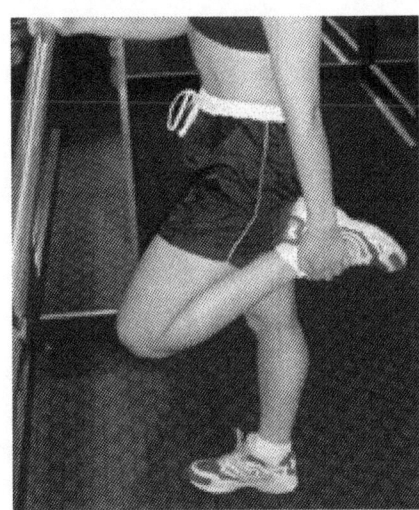 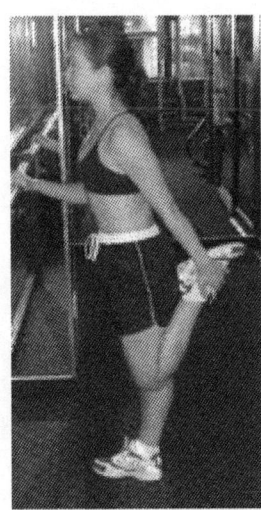

Figure 5.6   **Figure 5.7**

quadriceps. The whole process takes about thirty seconds. Then switch to the right quadriceps, and then stretch both the left and right sides again.

I'd like to digress for a moment and describe how I developed these stretches as an integrated routine. I was in the Colorado Rockies, on the second day of a week-long wildflower photography workshop. The summer before I had been in Yosemite National Park for a couple of days, hiking around and taking pictures of El Capitan, Bridalveil Falls, and Cathedral Rock. After a full day of hiking in Yosemite Valley I started to limp badly; an old knee injury began to act up. I really had trouble and the problem persisted for several days. I promptly forgot about it after I returned to New York (no one intentionally remembers pain one *used to* have), until the same pain shockingly reappeared after one day of hiking in the Rockies.

"Uh, oh", I thought. How was I going to enjoy my vacation? How was I going to get around with this debilitating knee pain? I worried all night and in the morning I had one of those welcome flashes of insight. My insight was to combine hamstring, calf, and quadriceps stretches as a routine. Previously I had recommended these stretches individually, piecemeal, to address isolated problem areas. I now had the realization that they were most effectively employed as a group, dealing with the lower extremity as a single unit. This made sense biomechanically and holistically, and was a revelation in terms of treatment.

In my specific instance, it was possible that by lengthening my leg musculature, my lower back and hip function would improve, alleviating a hypothetical stress on my knee. It worked! My knee pain and limp completely resolved. I had a great vacation and took some good pictures, and I had a new, effective treatment for a variety of lower back, hip, and knee disorders.

Over the years this stretching sequence has provided benefit to many patients. A lot of people have incorporated it as a regular part of their morning routine. I stretch this way before any physical activity, whether I'm running, lifting weights, riding my bike, or going to dance class.

Stretching prepares my body as a physical machine, enabling me to exercise full-out and have fun doing it.

There are many additional stretching routines, targeted to specific areas. An important one addresses the soft tissues around the hip joint, stretching muscles that flex the thigh on the hip and rotate the hip joint inward and outward. This stretch is done lying on your back, and it may be performed after the hamstring stretch. Let's stretch the left hip first. With the right leg straight and resting on the floor, gently bring the left knee toward your right shoulder, using your hands placed underneath the left knee. Angle the direction of pull so that you feel a stretch along the outside of the left thigh. This stretches the iliotibial band, a thin, long structure connecting the hip and the knee. Continue the stretch for fifteen or twenty seconds, replace the left leg on the floor, and stretch the right side. Repeat both sides.

The hip musculature can also be stretched in a seated position. We'll stretch the left side first. With your right knee bent and your right foot on the floor, place your hands underneath your left knee and bring it toward your left shoulder (Figure 5.8). Continue this stretch for ten or fifteen seconds. Then change the direction of stretch so that the left knee is being brought toward the right shoulder (Figure 5.9). Here you should feel a stretch along the outside of the left knee, stretching the iliotibial band.

Lastly, place your left foot on your right knee in cross-legged position and apply gentle downward pressure with your left hand on your left knee (Figure 5.10). Maintain this stretch for about ten seconds. This stretches the hip external rotators. Repeat the sequence on the right hip.

A useful stretch for the upper body addresses the latissimus dorsi and triceps. The latissimus is the large expanse of muscle on either side of the back which provides width and mass to the upper torso. It is active in various rowing motions. The triceps is the muscle on the back of the arm; it's function is to extend the elbow. The latissimus/triceps stretch may be done either sitting or standing. Let's stretch the left side first. Lift your left elbow so that your left arm is parallel to your head (your head is erect). Allow your left forearm to dangle, with your left hand resting near your right shoulder. This position of the forearm will allow the left arm to turn out slightly. Now, using the tips of your right index and middle fingers, apply a backward and centrally directed pressure to the center of the left elbow. You'll feel a stretch along the triceps and outer portion of the latissimus. Continue for ten or fifteen seconds and stretch the right side. Repeat both sides. This stretch also lengthens tight neck muscles.

To recap, stretching wakes up muscles that have been relatively asleep. Stretching lengthens muscles, allowing them to regain a more efficient configuration. Physiologically, local capillaries dilate, bringing increased blood flow to the muscles, warming them in the process. Now we're ready to exercise.

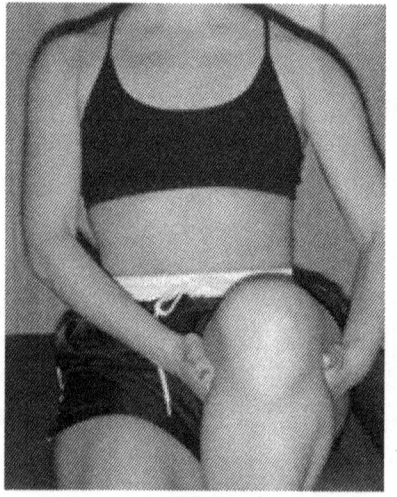

Figure 5.8

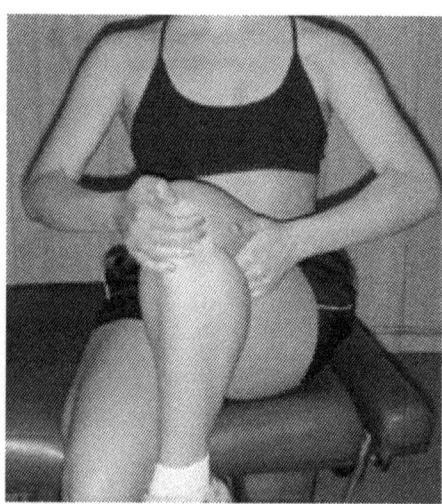

Figure 5.9

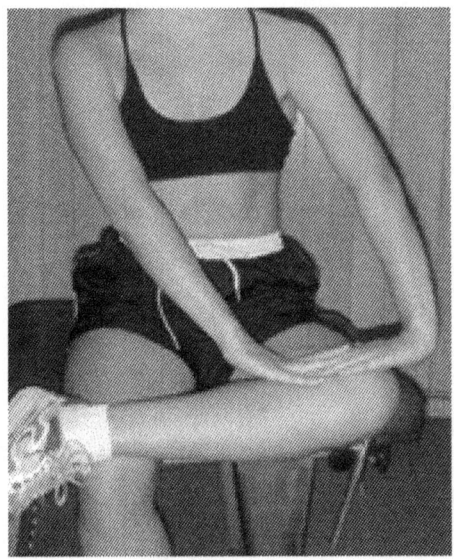

Figure 5.10

CHAPTER 6

▼

WEIGHT-TRAINING: DO YOU REALLY THINK I'M GOING TO LIFT THAT?

Lifting weights, "pumping iron", is one of the most useful and beneficial forms of exercise you could be doing. You could be doing lots of exercise-type activities, and if you weren't also lifting weights with some consistency your program wouldn't be complete. Weight-training is useful for anybody, of any age. You might be thinking, "Yeah, right. I'm already doing plenty. What do I want to fool around with weights for? I don't want to get big muscles. I've heard you can hurt yourself lifting weights." And possibly more words to that effect. What exactly am I suggesting?

First, some full disclosure. I've been lifting weights, on and off but mostly on, since 1984. I heard about weightlifting from my friend Stan, a classmate at chiropractic school. This particular conversation took place about two years after I had stopped dancing. I had been establishing my chiropractic practice, and hadn't made time to find a suitable activity to replace the intensity of dance class. Having been at peak condition, I was then less than peak and not happy about it. Stan talked about lifting weights and how much fun it was. Of course, I remembered Charles Atlas and Steve Reeves and had watched powerlifting competitions on TV. What I didn't know about was the tremendous physiologic benefit of weight-training; nor did I have any inkling of the how-to's of it, the science of weight-training. But Stan's enthusiasm was infectious, and I went to a local gym and had my first few workouts with weights.

I was profoundly sore after those early sessions, indicating my lack of conditioning relative to that particular activity. Postexercise soreness is due to a build-up of lactic acid. Since the muscles aren't well-trained there's a dearth of capillaries, and the metabolic end-products of muscle work are removed slowly. Once training progresses capillary circulation is extended and lactic acid is removed quickly. So a "charley horse" or muscle soreness is normal and not to be feared or avoided. As it turned out, I loved lifting weights. I loved everything about going to the gym: the tactile sensations of the dumbbells and barbells and the weight plates, the challenge of doing increased repetitions and lifting heavier loads, actually *seeing* the muscle work in the mirror, the swelling of the tissues and the distention of the veins. But you already knew I was exercise-crazy.

I dived into the subject and started reading weight-training magazines. By great good fortune I met two enthusiastic gym assistants (this was before there were personal trainers) who graciously shared their knowledge and expertise. Over the course of several years I learned a whole catalog of exercises and routines, had many injuries, and managed to gain something from each one (mostly how to exercise hard and *not* injure myself). I also learned something about *process,* which has application to other fields as well. In weight-training, what works, works. In other words, a system of exercising that works for me does just that: it works for me.

There is a universe of systems and methods about how to train. Frequently, proponents of a particular system or style believe their method is best. However, if you selected one gym member from twelve top gyms and had each one describe his training system, twelve completely different styles of training might be recounted. Which one would be right for you? The answer would be: which one *works* for you? In other words, which system provides the best workout, the most efficient strength gains for you? Which one is the most fun, has you look forward to going to the gym, is most suited to your body and temperament?

Having explored a number of systems, evaluating them from the point of view of *results*, I concluded that no system has universal application. My body type is ectomorphic—long and slender. Is the style of training that's best for me also effective for a mesomorphic body type, one that's relatively broader with more potential muscle mass? Not necessarily. Will my workout routine be effective for a person with an endomorphic body type, one with a higher proportion of fat and a bigger abdomen? Probably not.

The best workouts are individualized. The best workouts take principles from many systems, applying them where needed. What will work for me? What is optimal for my body? What tested principles can I apply that will be effective in achieving my goals of physical fitness? Will I see benefits both in the short-term and the long-term? Will I have fun doing it so that I will do it again? These are the questions we'll address as we investigate this marvelous tool: weight-training.

First, let's consider what makes weight-training so effective. Yes, it makes muscles stronger and bigger, but really, what's the use of that? The benefit of weight-training is that it teaches the body how to handle loads under varying and frequently difficult circumstances. I know that sounds pretty clinical, rather dry. Said another way, weight-training prepares you to develop more skills, have more fun, and expand your participation in a variety of sports, such as tennis, golf, skiing, rollerblading, running, biking, and swimming. In fact, there's no sport in which weight-training won't make a difference. Weight-training provides a framework in which you can excel and lowers the chance of sports-related injury. Let's look at how these things are accomplished. Then we'll talk about actual weight-training methods and how to apply them.

When you lift a weight you're lifting it through an arc of motion. If you're doing a biceps curl, for example, the elbow travels from a starting position of about 5 degrees of elbow bend to a finishing position of about 125 degrees, thus describing an arc of motion of about 120 degrees. If you're doing a "lat pulldown" the shoulder joint travels from starting position of about 170 degrees (almost parallel to the torso) to a finishing position of about 50 degrees, again describing an arc of motion of about 120 degrees. If you're doing quad extensions, the knee travels from a starting position of about 90 degrees of flexion to a finishing position of about 0 degrees of flexion, describing an arc of motion of about 90 degrees.

The joint or joints involved in an exercise are supporting a load throughout the joint's range of motion. Torques are applied to the joint structures during the entire movement. Muscles, tendons, and ligaments resist the mechanical stresses, and muscles and bones move the weight smoothly through the arc of motion. This process gets a little more difficult with each successive repetition. You know this—the weight you're moving feels heavier the more reps you do. More muscle fibers are recruited to assist in moving the weight. Here's where the "training" part of weight-training comes in.

Increased repetitions require the participation of increased numbers of muscle fibers. The ability to recruit those additional muscle fibers necessitates increased communication between the nerves activating those fibers and the muscle fibers themselves. In other words, if previously one particular nerve activated ten fibers in its potential network, now, several repetitions later, that same nerve must activate fifteen fibers. At the end of the set, that nerve might be activating twenty fibers. The nerve is being trained to be more effective, to extend its range of influence.

Also, contraction of increased numbers of muscle fibers requires an increased supply of raw materials. More oxygen is needed; more glucose is needed. There is a build-up of metabolic end-products which must be swept away. New capillaries are constructed to supply the expanding metabolic demands of the muscle tissue. Thus, the entire muscular system is being trained in efficient performance: nerves, capillaries, and muscle fibers all improve in efficiency. This miraculous result occurs on a cellular level when you lift dumbbells or barbells or work on a piece of equipment for increasing numbers of repetitions over time.

Another physiologic benefit of lifting weights relates to proprioception, the body's awareness of its position in space. The tangible result of training the proprioceptive system is a reduction in frequency of injuries in your other sports. The proprioceptive system is composed of specialized nerve endings located in muscles, tendons, ligaments, and joints; various nerve pathways; and the parts of the brain devoted to balance and coordinated movement. The system relays information concerning muscle action, the speed and angular momentum of movement of a joint, and the position of a joint at a specific moment in time. Proprioception makes coordinated movement possible. Weight-training trains the proprioceptive system in balancing weight and moving loads throughout a joint's range of motion. Many joint/muscle/tendon systems are brought into play during a specific exercise; therefore many links in the proprioceptive system are trained simultaneously. It is an efficient process.

The proprioceptive system answers questions such as "how much force needs to be exerted in these specific muscles to move these bones through this particular arc of motion". Said another way, "What precise forces need to be produced to pick up this pen and write with it?" Or, "What forces are needed to brake my rollerblades at the bottom of the hill?" Or, "What forces do I apply to the steering wheel and accelerator pedal to maintain traction across this icy road?" If you had to make a conscious decision for each subtle movement, nothing would get done. Only the most basic actions would be possible. The proprioceptive system is an important component of all our daily activities. Proprioceptive training makes your joints *smart.*

Athletic activity often requires extreme movement. Unplanned, unforeseen situations occur which require an instantaneous response. Fine muscular adjustments become necessary to maintain balance, avoid an accident, or make a shot. A precisely trained proprioceptive system is one key to athletic performance. Performance gains result from instruction, repetition, and as has become evident in the last fifteen years or so, weight-training.

Let's look at injury prevention. Tennis elbow is a common injury among people who work during the week and also play tennis. The workday doesn't prepare you physically to engage in this sport. Significant forces may be generated at the elbow during a powerful serve or strong backhand return. What is the preparation for properly withstanding these forces so that there is no soft tissue damage? If there has been no preparation, injury is probable over time. If preparation has consisted of tennis lessons, the likelihood of injury is reduced: you have been trained, to a greater or lesser degree, in the biomechanics of the sport. If preparation has included both instruction and weight-training, the likelihood of injury is even further reduced. In the latter case, the elbow has been trained to withstand significant loads throughout its full range of motion. It can undergo the stress of high-end forces developed during a vigorous game of tennis without sustaining an injury: the elbow can bend but not break. Weight-training allows you to play hard with a greatly reduced risk of injury.

Ankle sprains are another common injury whose incidence can be reduced through specific exercise. In Manhattan, where I live, the city streets undergo constant renovation. Heavy traffic and wet winter weather create potholes; curbs are uneven due to use and abuse; unexpected objects of various sizes lying in the street may be suddenly encountered. There are many opportunities to "turn over" an ankle in Manhattan. Some people suffer ankle sprains because they twisted an ankle stepping off a curb; others have no problem after a similar twist. What's the difference?

The difference might lie in the noninjured ankle's ability to withstand unusually heavy loads in extreme positions, at the limits of its normal range of motion. Such an ability is one of the benefits of weight-training. The injured ankle, presumably untrained, compensates poorly or inefficiently to the unusual, unexpected, extreme mechanical load and deformation of the twisted position. The soft tissues in this ankle are not as plastic as those in the trained ankle, whose soft tissues can deform and return to normal within a broader range of performance.

A third example relates to injury of the rotator cuff, the sheath of muscle that covers the shoulder and elevates and rotates the arm. The rotator cuff may be injured acutely in a specific activity or it may deteriorate over time. Due to the design of the shoulder, the blood supply to the rotator cuff is compromised every time the arm is fully elevated to the side. This temporary loss of blood supply creates a "critical zone" within the rotator cuff tendon. The tissues in the critical zone may eventually weaken or fray. Microtears may develop into chronic injury. Weight-training provides an efficient counter to this process, in that collateral circulation is built up in response to the physiologic stress of lifting weights. Over time, a greater supply of blood reaches the tissues of the rotator cuff, countering the ischemic (decrease in blood supply) effects and diminishing the likelihood of chronic injury.

Should we lift weights so that we can prevent injuries? Yes, and also let's lift weights so we can excel in our sporting activities, playing as hard as we want for as many years as we want.

I'd like to note a few caveats before we look at how to train. People often say they don't want to start weight-training because they don't want to "get big". Certainly, some people will build muscle mass more quickly than do others. The first stages of weight-training establish efficient connections between nerve fibers and muscle fibers. Each nerve fiber learns to send electrical signals to more muscle fibers. Initially the muscle mass you already have becomes more efficient; only after these connections are saturated is it necessary to add more muscle fibers. Also, you only get *really* big if you are lifting heavy weight and are in the gym six times a week. Weight-training three or four times a week with moderate weight will add shapely muscle mass without creating a bulky look. Also, a well-designed, comprehensive program will lead to overall strength gains and an attractive physique.

In contrast, other people will try to hit the weights hard, doing too much too soon, and hurt themselves. Weight-training is almost always a go-slow, build-over-time process. Forcing the process, ignoring the facts of physiology, will usually result in injury. Then training is set back a number of weeks, it's boring, you're frustrated, all the rest. I know. I've had these injuries, a *long* list. For years I was a smart aleck. Hey, I was a dancer. I *know* my body. But I didn't know weight-training. I'll admit it took way too long for me to get it, to finally learn patience. Fortunately, I can share my experience. Your training will simply be fun, valuable, and injury-free.

A useful method for beginners is to start with five basic exercises for the upper body: bench press, lat pulldown, shoulder press, biceps curl, and triceps curl. I'll explain each term as we go along. This group of five exercises works the chest, back, shoulders, and arms. Start with the amount of weight with which you can do a set of eight repetitions comfortably, without straining at the end of the set. There should be effort involved in completing the set, but not strain. If possible, do three sets of eight repetitions each for each exercise. If you can do one set of eight, a second set of seven reps, and a final set of five or six reps, that's fine too. Your strength and coordination will improve and so will the numbers of reps. In this early training, one goal is to do three sets of eight reps each with a moderately challenging weight. You'll get there.

It's never too early to talk about form, so let's start right here. Many things can go wrong when lifting weights, most of them relating to poor or incorrect form. With good form your weight is balanced on two legs, or it's distributed evenly across your buttocks if you're sitting, or across your pelvis and back if you're lying on your back. Concentrate on using the correct muscle for the particular exercise. The main muscle used in an exercise is called the *prime mover*. If you're doing a bench press, the prime mover is the pectoralis major. When doing shoulder presses, the prime mover is the deltoid. The latissimus dorsi is the prime mover for lat pulldowns. Visualize the prime mover working during the exercise. Visualize the muscle's origin and insertion and see the muscle contracting as you do the repetition. Visualizing the activity of the prime mover will eliminate a good portion of strain in supporting muscles. These supporting muscles are the *stabilizers* of the movement. It's easy to rely on supporting muscles when lifting weights. These stabilizing structures, for the most part, are *postural* muscles. Basically, postural muscles keep the body erect; they maintain an upright position or posture. They are, in effect, antigravity muscles. Postural muscles include the trapezius, hamstrings, and the erector spinae, a complex group of short, medium-length, and long muscles that support the spine.

Since the postural antigravity muscles are stabilizers, they participate in the process of lifting weights. This represents natural, coordinated activity. However, it's easy to *substitute* postural contractions for prime mover contractions, and attempt to lift or move the weight primarily by using the stabilizers. This substitution pattern can take over when the prime mover begins to fatigue, and injury may result. You strain a neck or back muscle because you were inadvertently using those muscles to lift the weight, rather than using the biceps, deltoid, or pectorals.

The large majority of these postural muscle strains can be avoided simply by *paying attention*. Visualize the prime movers doing the work. There will be stabilizer support, but it is *support*. Check the position of your shoulders. The shoulders should not be elevated (if they are, then the trapezius muscles are contracting inappropriately). The shoulder girdles should be resting on the rib cage even though work is being done. Are you tightening the central muscles of your back? Of course, these muscles do contract for support, but are you initiating or maintaining the movement of the weight by causing these spinal muscles to contract? Movement is initiated and maintained by the prime mover. Now, there's naturally more effort being done by the stabilizing muscles during the final repetitions of a set, but make sure that your body is not distorting, your body weight is evenly distributed, and you're still concentrating on using the prime mover.

Injuries commonly occur on the last repetition of a set, when the muscle being worked is fatigued. You want to do one more rep, you don't want to give up, you're close to setting a new standard, you said you were going to do it, or whatever. You will do that last rep: any considerations you might have had regarding proper form are forgotten and you strain and grunt and contort and move that weight one more time. However, the prime mover isn't doing the lifting on this last, gasping rep. Accessory muscles, stabilizers, and postural muscles are doing the lifting and muscle strain is likely.

How do you avoid injury at the end of a set? The last few reps *are* very important; be sure to do them with strict form. If you can't move the weight through your full range of motion without contorting, don't complete that rep. Rest for a minute and start the next set. Maintaining good form will keep you injury-free and simultaneously train your body in efficient performance—this is what it takes to do this, this is what it takes to do that, this much contraction of these muscles is needed to support that movement, and so on. Your body's machinery—the muscles, tendons, ligaments, and bones—and the computational network that organizes that activity—the nervous system—are trained, retrained, and refined for maximum performance each time you go to the gym.

OK. We've been paying attention to good form. Good form will guide all our activities in the gym. Let's start our first training session with the bench press. Lie on your back on the bench so that your sternum (breastbone) is directly under the barbell. Most barbells have a thin circumferential groove on each side, about eighteen or so inches from the center. Place your little fingers around these grooves for optimal positioning. Your feet can be on the floor; however, your back is very supported if your knees are bent and your heels are on the bench at the end of the bench (Figure 6.1).

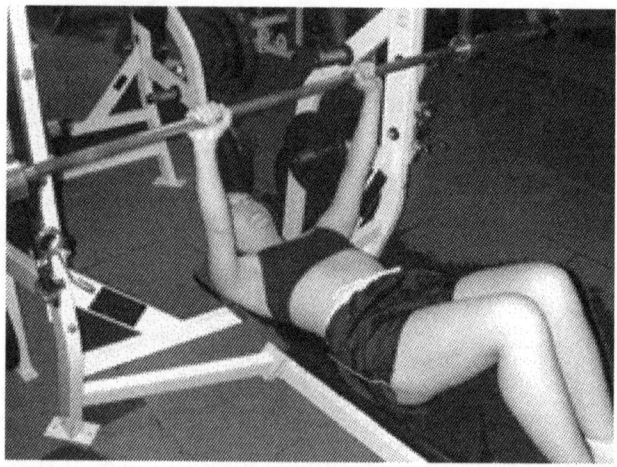

Figure 6.1

Straighten your arms, lifting the barbell off the rack. Lower the barbell to your sternum (Figure 6.2) and raise it back up, straightening your elbows. Move purposefully, with moderate speed, not too fast and not too slow. Don't forcefully straighten or lock your elbows at the conclusion of the repetition.

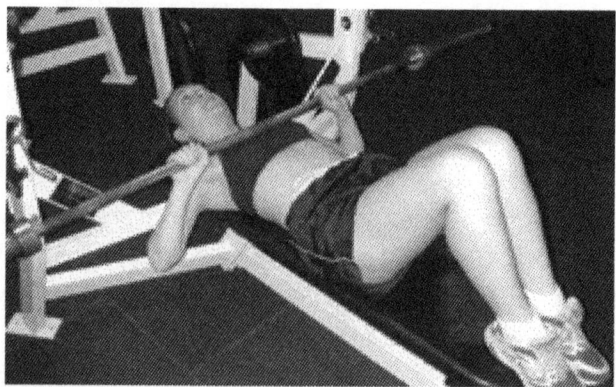

Figure 6.2

Be sure to keep your lower back flat on the bench during the entire repetition. Avoid arching your lower back (this is a violation of form and potentially dangerous). How much weight should you use as a beginner? The longest barbell, an Olympic bar, weighs forty-five pounds. Most men and some women could start their first beginner sets with this weight alone. A somewhat shorter barbell, found in most gyms, weighs thirty pounds; the "E-Z curl" bar, a short bar with an angled middle portion, weighs twenty pounds. Start with these lighter bars if the Olympic bar is too heavy to do eight repetitions. Stronger individuals or those who have lifted weights in the past may start by pressing sixty-five or eighty-five pounds (placing one or two ten-pound plates on each side). Remember to place a clip or weight-lock on each side if you're adding plates. If you can, do three sets of eight repetitions each. We'll talk about varying sets, reps, and weights after we've discussed the basic exercises.

The lat pulldown machine is next. All things being equal, if you have a choice between using free weights and using a machine for a particular exercise, choose the free weights (barbells and dumbbells). When you work with free weights, both the prime mover and other accessory and stabilizing muscles are being trained simultaneously. There is more result per unit of effort. When you use a machine, more work is done by the prime mover and less by other supporting muscles. Machines are relatively easier to use. Machines are a great tool and can be used to advantage as a means of varying one's workout. But in general, given a choice, use free weights. For some exercises, such as the lat pulldown, the machine version is the only choice. This is a powerful exercise, one that provides excellent conditioning, shaping, and strength gains.

"Lat" stands for latissimus dorsi, a broad sheet of muscle which extends from the mid-back, crosses the upper/outer back, and inserts on the upper arm. Developing the lat creates a broad "V" across the upper back. The lat pulldown is performed in a seated position. Your knees go under the padded rollers at the front of the seat and should just touch their undersurface. Adjust the height of the rollers if necessary, stand up, and grasp either end of the bar. Each little finger should be near the end of the straight portion of the bar, just before the bar bends on either side. Sit down with a steady motion, drawing the bar down with you. You should be seated with your arms raised overhead, holding onto the bar. This is the starting position (Figure 6.3).

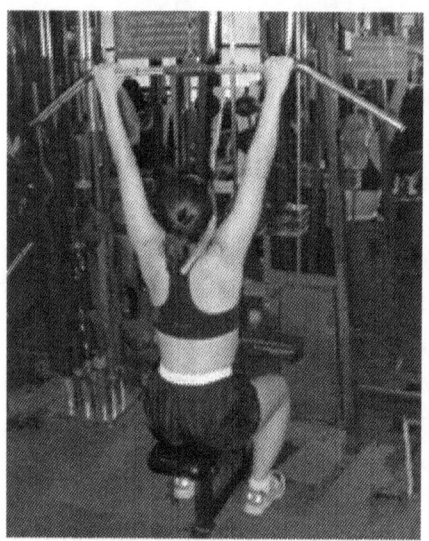 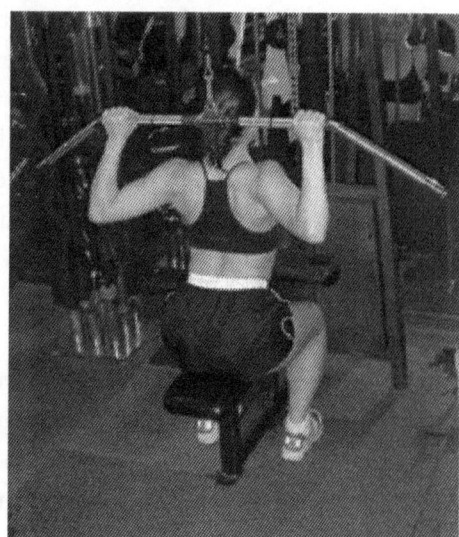

Figure 6.3   **Figure 6.4**

It's a good idea to *prestretch* in this exercise. Prestretching can be done for some exercises; it lengthens the muscle that's about to do some work, so that more work can be done with the same effort. Prestretch here by letting the shoulders elevate: let the weight of the bar naturally drag the shoulders upward. Where they come to rest is the prestretched position. Pull the bar down smoothly and evenly, slightly behind your neck, until it touches your upper back (Figure 6.4). (In a variation, bring the bar down in front of your neck.) Then release, raising the bar smoothly and evenly until you return to the overhead position. This is one repetition. Prestretch to start the next rep. Avoid swinging your torso back and forth to move the bar: the movement is initiated by the lats and, secondarily, the biceps. Also, avoid using your neck muscles as much as possible: they are involved, *but* attempt to minimize this by concentrating on the lats and biceps. Beginners can start with anywhere from ten to forty pounds (one to four plates on a typical lat machine).

Next is the shoulder press. This can be done seated on a bench with dumbbells or seated on a specially designed bench with a rack for military presses, which are shoulder presses done with a barbell. Dumbbells are optimal in the early stages of training because each arm gets to carry its own load, each arm is trained individually. Later, either dumbbells or barbells are fine. With dumbbells, it's best to sit on an incline bench with the tilting part upright, so that your upper back is supported by the upright part of the bench. Grasp a dumbbell in either hand and raise your hands overhead by straightening your elbows. This is the beginning position (Figure 6.5).

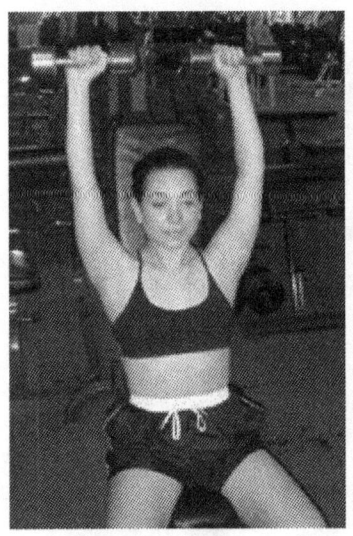

Figure 6.5

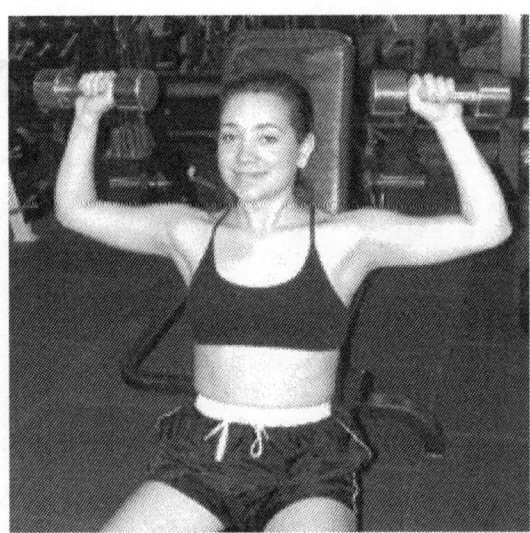

Figure 6.6

Lower the dumbbells to shoulder level and return to the overhead position (Figure 6.6). This is one repetition. Men who have never trained before can start with eight-pound dumbbells. Women who have never trained before can start with three- or five-pound dumbbells. If you've trained before but haven't in a while, start with ten-pounders. It's a hard exercise. Don't elevate the shoulder girdles during the pressing part of the rep; keep the shoulders on the rib cage. Press the dumbbells overhead by using the shoulder *muscles,* not by rotating the shoulder blades.

Now we'll do two arm exercises, one for the biceps and one for the triceps. The biceps flexes the elbow; the triceps extends the elbow. An optimal biceps exercise is the incline biceps curl, done with dumbbells. Sit on an incline bench with the incline peg at hole #5, providing an incline of about 25 degrees from the vertical. Grasping a dumbbell in each hand, alternately curl one dumbbell and then the other, bringing the dumbbell toward your shoulder, fully flexing the elbow on each curl (Figures 6.7 and 6.8).

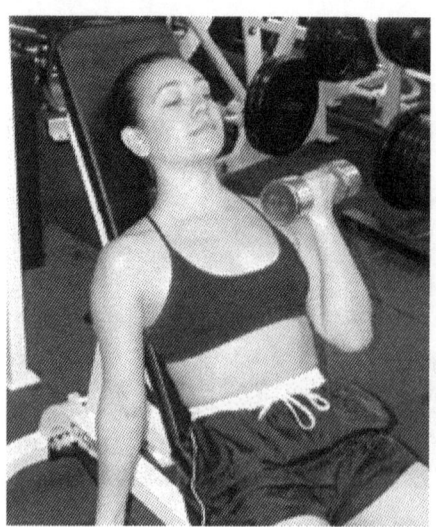
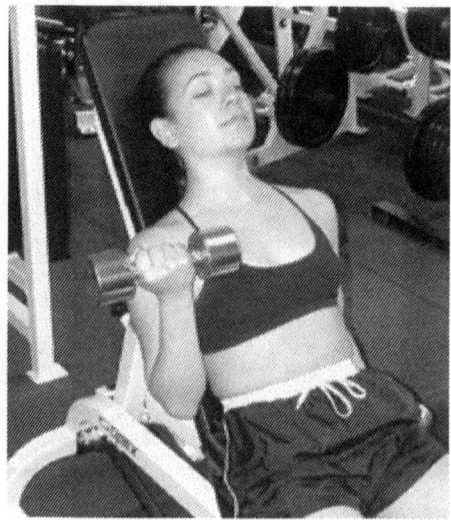

Figure 6.7   **Figure 6.8**

Avoid swinging the dumbbell; the motion is smooth and steady. Also, as much as possible, avoid lifting the dumbbell with the shoulder to perform the first thirty degrees of curling motion. Use the biceps throughout the exercise. A good beginning weight for a woman would be five-pound dumbbells. A good beginning weight for a man would be ten-pounders. Remember, it's not the heaviness of the weight that counts. It's the quality of your concentration and the strictness of your form that produce strength gains and excellent long-term results.

The triceps extension is next. We'll work with the same machine we used for lat pulldowns, but we'll be standing instead of sitting. Stand facing the machine so that the bar is in front of you. Place your hands on either side of the center of the bar, resting your thumbs on top of the bar, and bring the bar down to about the level of your sternum (Figure 6.9). Keeping your elbows close to your sides, press the bar all the way down by straightening your elbows (Figure 6.10). Then allow the bar to return to its original position at the level of your sternum. This is one repetition. A good starting weight for a woman would be one plate (ten pounds); a good starting weight for a man would be two plates. Bring the bar down in a steady and smooth motion; don't force your elbows into a straightened position.

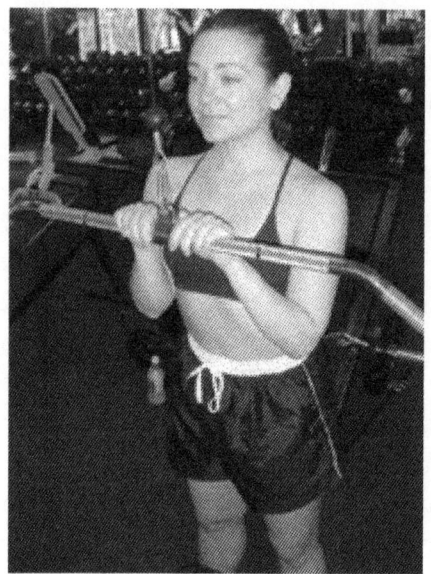 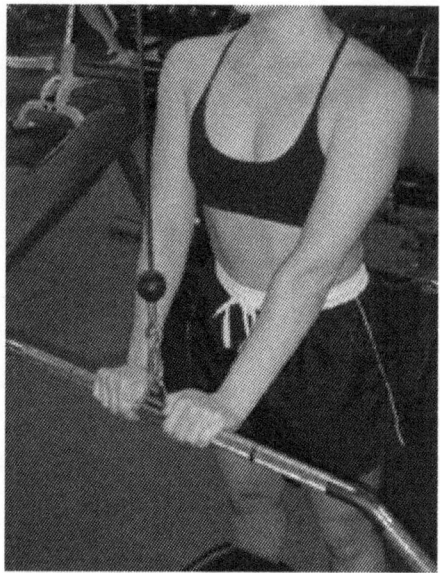

Figure 6.9   **Figure 6.10**

Next is the back extension, a simple, but critical, exercise designed to strengthen the lower back. Most gyms have the small piece of equipment used in this exercise. One version of this "Roman chair" has a saddle which supports your pelvis and two rollers under which you place your ankles, stabilizing your legs in a horizontal position. Your torso, arms, and head hang freely over the front of the saddle. Another version has an angled foot plate at its base. You hook your heels against the top edge of the foot plate, your thighs are supported by a wider angled plate, and you hang your torso over the top edge. These setups may sound pretty primitive; they're basic, simple structures, throwbacks to the earliest days of weight-training.

The exercise is quite straightforward: With your torso hanging toward the ground, place your fingertips on either side of your skull with your elbows flared out to the sides (Figure 6.11). Using your lower back muscles, elevate your torso until it forms a straight line with your buttocks and legs: if you were standing, this would be an upright position (Figure 6.12).

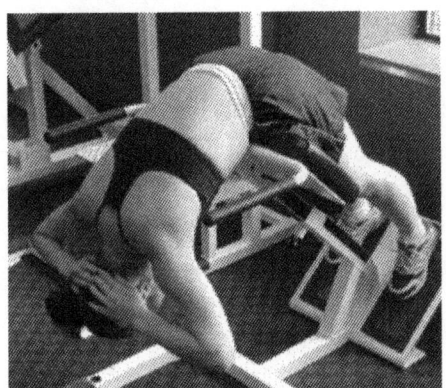 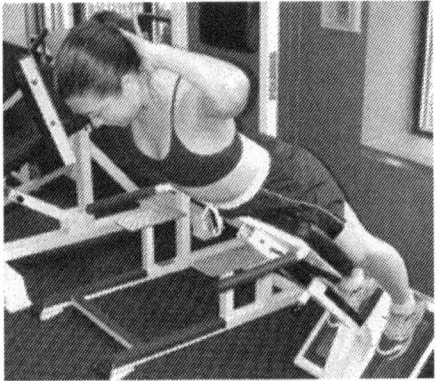

Figure 6.11   **Figure 6.12**

Avoid going past this straightened position into one that arches the lower back: such a hyperextended position can create stress in the lumbar spinal joints. Back extensions are difficult if you've never done them: start with two sets of six repetitions and build up to three sets of twelve. It is normal to experience lower back tightening during the course of this exercise. We almost never specifically address these back extensor muscles; in most people, these muscles are weak and need to be trained. The tightness is a normal consequence of muscle work and will recede later in the day.

The last exercise in our beginning routine is for the abdominal muscles. I know, you were hoping I would skip this part. I admit that it's easy to ignore abdominal training. If you're running, abdominal work needs to be specifically added: you get home after a run, flop down on your exercise mat, and work your abs. Sure. Mostly this doesn't happen, and you achieve great aerobic fitness and have weak lower abdominals (the upper abs are worked somewhat during running). This may result in lower back problems later on. Or, you lift weights, work hard, and then at the end of your workout you remember: Oh, right, what about doing some stomach exercises? Well, it's much easier to say, "I'll do it next time" and head for the showers. Again, the upper abdominals are worked during weight-training; the lower abdominals are not. Lower back problems are a possibility when abdominal training depends on your mood.

It definitely takes something *extra* to train your abdominals consistently. I propose that abdominal training will get done on a steady basis if you start your workouts with the *intention* of doing stomach exercises at the end. You've built it in to your mental program for that day and when it's time to do them, you do them. You're intentional about it rather than having it as an afterthought. After a while the abdominal work is just another component of your routine.

There are many benefits to training your abdominals. Looking good could easily be at the top of the list. How many infomercials are targeted to the "sagging tummy" population? If you sit for most of the day, your abdominals are getting weaker, muscle tone is being lost, and a slight roundness is developing. The only way to reverse this process is to do abdominal exercises. The main physiologic benefit relates to support for the lower back. As with hamstring and quadriceps tightness, a person could be perfectly normal and develop lower back pain because his abdominals were weak. The abdominal muscles support the weight of the abdominal contents: the liver, stomach, pancreas, intestines, and the rest. They also resist the mechanical tendency for the lumbar spine to hyperextend, helping to support the normal lumbar lordosis and avoiding a swayback. Weak abdominals are implicated in lower back pain: it's a direct relationship.

Thus, strong, trained abdominals are to be desired; the downside is that abdominals are notoriously difficult to train. Mistakes and misconceptions abound in training routines. I consulted with a patient last week concerning an acute lower back injury she sustained at the gym. She's in her late forties and in great shape. We talked about her routine and how she injured herself, and I learned that she did her abdominal routine *first*, before she did any other exercises. Also, she did exercises for her middle abdominals, her abdominal obliques, and her lower abdominals, but she did the lower abdominal exercises *last*.

There are two major training errors here. The abdominals help to support the body's weight and are active whenever you are standing, and may be active when you are sitting if you intentionally utilize them. Therefore, they function as supporting muscles during most weight-training exercises and are *needed* in that capacity. If they are trained first, before doing anything else, then they are not available for their supporting function. Two things will occur. You will not be able to train as effectively because you worked your abdominals first. Also, your lower back is at risk because you have fatigued your abdominals and are now lifting weights. Abdominal exercises are done last because these muscles are needed to support most other exercises.

The abdominal muscles consist of four groups: the lower, oblique, middle, and upper abdominals. The oblique abdominals (the internal and external obliques) are arranged in a cross-hatched pattern on either side of your torso. The lower abdominals are trained first because they're the weakest. If you train them at the end of the routine, as my patient was doing, there's not much strength available and other muscles, such as lower back muscles, may be recruited to perform the movement. Lower back strain can result. After the lower abs are worked, the obliques and middle abs are done next, in whichever order. The upper abs are done last.

Let's start with the lower abs. Lie on your back on an exercise mat. Place your hands, palms down, at your sides near your waist or buttocks. Contract your abdominals slightly so that your upper back and head are elevated five or so degrees off the floor. With legs straight (or with a slight knee bend), elevate both legs about six inches. This is the starting position for leg raises (Figure 6.13). Raise the legs to a ninety-degree position (perpendicular to the floor; Figure 6.14) and lower them to just six inches off the floor. This is one repetition.

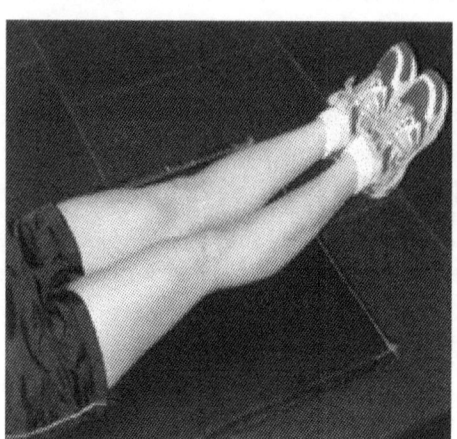

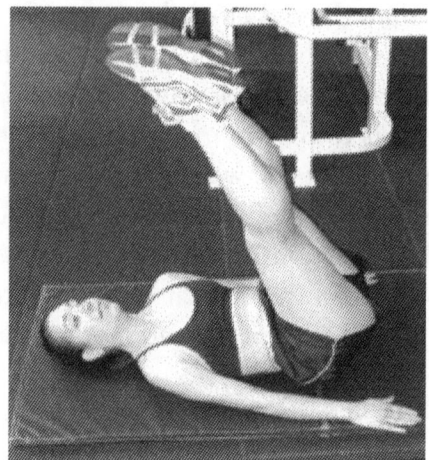

Figure 6.13   **Figure 6.14**

Start with a set of eight repetitions. Rest for fifteen seconds and do another set of eight. Build over four to six weeks to two sets of twenty-five reps. This is a difficult exercise for beginners, since untrained lower abdominals are generally pretty weak. Any exercise specifically designed for the lower abdominals would be difficult; this exercise is safe and efficient. Be sure you're not arching your lower back during either the raising or lowering part of the repetition. Keep the lower back flat on the mat.

When you can do two sets of twenty-five leg raises, you're ready to use a more difficult exercise: leg raises with a pelvic lift. Here, the leg raise part of the repetition is the same; when you get to the ninety-degree position, lift the pelvis straight up in the air—this is an elevated pelvic tilt—then lower the pelvis to the floor and lower the legs to six inches above the floor. This is one repetition. Adding the pelvic raise causes the lower abdominals to do more work during each repetition. Start with two sets of twelve to fifteen repetitions; build to two sets of twenty-five reps.

When you can do that many leg raise/pelvic lifts, you're ready to begin advanced lower abdominal exercises. These exercises use a piece of equipment called a leg-raise unit, which is a vertical frame with two foot plates and two horizontal arm rests. You step onto the foot supports and place your forearms on the arm rests. Your forearms support your body weight during the exercises. The first routine involves leg swings. The knees are bent at about seventy degrees. Without swinging your torso, swing your legs into the air, bringing your knees toward your chest, and lower your legs back down to a neutral hanging position. This is one repetition. Do a set of six repetitions, rest fifteen seconds, and do another set of six. Build to two sets of fifteen.

The second advanced abdominal exercise is called knee-ups. Raise your knees as high as you can, bending at the hips to perform this motion, and lower the thighs to a neutral, straight position, maintaining the knee bend. Start with two sets of six and build to two sets of fifteen. Or, you can add difficulty by doing one set of leg swings and then, without resting, doing a set of knee-ups. Build to two sets each of fifteen leg swings/fifteen knee-ups.

Now we'll train the abdominal obliques. Lie on your back on the mat, bend your right leg to ninety degrees (keeping the right foot on the mat), and place your left foot across your right knee, allowing the left knee to open into a cross-legged position (Figure 6.15). Place your right fingers on the back of your head, keeping your elbow away from your body, and extend your left arm on the mat at about a thirty-degree angle from your torso. Raise your head and right side of your torso off the floor, bringing your right elbow toward your left knee.

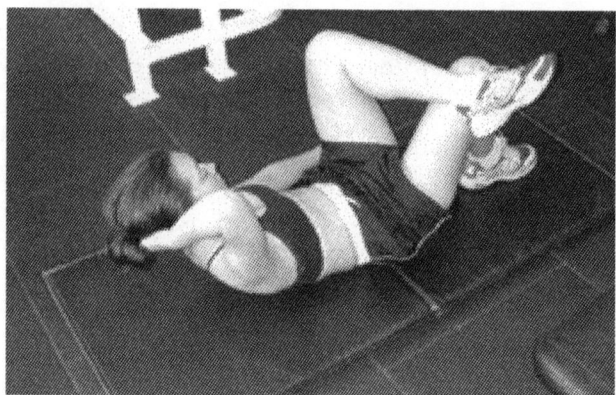

Figure 6.15

Lower almost, but not quite, back to the floor. This is one repetition. You're not going too far here, there's not much elevation of your head and right shoulder in the beginning. You might only raise up an inch or so, angling your right elbow toward your left knee. When your abdominals are more trained you're still only elevating several inches off the floor. So, don't be discouraged by a minimal amount of movement. That's all there is right now. Do fifteen reps and then do the left side, reversing the position. In the exercise for the left obliques, you're attempting to bring your left elbow toward your right knee. Build to twenty-five reps for each side.

Next are the middle abdominals (these are the muscles that, when developed, create the "washboard" appearance). Both feet are on the floor for this routine, with both knees bent to ninety degrees. Place your fingertips on either side of your head with your elbows out to the sides. Lift your head and shoulders off the floor in a curling motion by contracting your middle abs, aiming your sternum toward your knees (Figure 6.16). Again, you're not elevating too far off the floor, maybe an inch or so. That's fine; you're training your abdominals. Eventually you'll elevate several inches, curling toward your knees. Do ten or twelve of these "crunches" to start; build to thirty-five or forty.

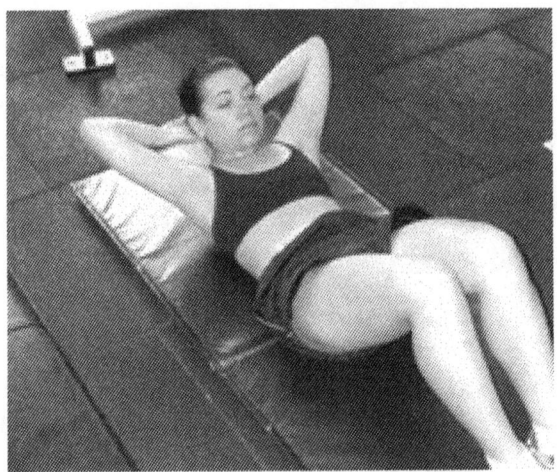

Figure 6.16

The last piece of this four-part abdominal routine is for the upper abs (the top layer of the washboard). Position your hips and knees so that your thighs are straight up (perpendicular to the floor) and your knees are bent at ninety degrees (calves are parallel to the floor). Place your fingertips on either side of your head with your elbows out to the sides. Curl your head and shoulders off the floor, this time aiming your sternum at an angle between the ceiling and your knees. This is an angled upward motion; you should feel the contraction in your upper abdominals. There will be little movement in the beginning. Start with ten or twelve and build to thirty-five or forty.

Beginners may experience neck discomfort or even strain in the early phases of abdominal training. I have recommended abdominal exercises to patients who have said, "Oh, no, I can't do those. They hurt my neck." This difficulty can be avoided. A beginner may strain neck muscles if he's using his neck to initiate the movement. The abdominals are weak and to achieve some movement the beginner will recruit postural muscles of the neck to raise the upper torso off the ground. Be sure you're *not* recruiting neck muscles when you do these exercises. Concentrate on the abdominals; *visualize* the muscles you are exercising. Make those muscles do the work. Remind yourself to disengage the neck muscles and you will not suffer neck strain.

I admit this abdominal training sounds like a lot of work. Actually, the whole routine, all four parts, takes only ten minutes. In the beginning it is hard work, in the sense that your abs are weak and the exercises are tough. After a week or so you get in the groove and develop some kinesiologic sense of how the exercises are done—what part goes where, how to move this part or that part—and the routine gets easier. You develop a flatter abdomen, which looks great and provides a constant sense of accomplishment: Hey! Check out those abs! And, of course, strong abdominals support all of the body's mechanical activities. With respect to lower back injury, pain is managed much more effectively when there is underlying abdominal fitness. In my experience, episodes are less frequent and recovery is facilitated when a person is well-conditioned.

OK. We've been in the gym for about four weeks, going twice or three times each week. We've built up to three sets each for the five basic upper body exercises and we're doing the lower back extensions and the abdominal routine each time we train. Let's consider other exercises and training routines, other things that can be done in the gym. First let's look at exercises for the lower body. The major muscle groups are the quadriceps (front of the thigh), hamstrings (back of the thigh), and gastrocnemius/soleus (calves). These are all quite easy to train.

The most important lower body exercise is the squat. The squat, that venerable, mythic exercise, is in itself practically a complete weight-training routine. When you do a set of squats you're training the calves, quadriceps, hamstrings, buttocks, and lower back: in other words, the entire lower body is being trained by one exercise. Also, interestingly, there is a built-in cross-training effect with squats. Many people report an increase in upper body strength and tone after adding squats to their weekly weight routine.

How do you perform this miracle exercise? With strict attention to form. For a long while, squats were considered risky because of reported injuries to the lower back and knees. However, squatting itself was not the culprit; injuries were due to poor instruction and poor form. In a well-done squat, the head is tilted very slightly upward; the abdomen is active and strong; the lower back is flat, not arched; and the feet are hip-width apart and facing forward or slightly turned out. Also, the squat involves a knee bend to about ninety degrees, so that the thighs are parallel to the floor; and the knees are oriented over the first or second toe, angling neither inward nor outward. In the past, people squatted all the way down (you may still see people doing this), creating an acute knee angulation with increased stresses at the knee. Arching the lower back is often necessary to recover from this deep knee bend to a standing position. Both knee and lower back injuries are possible due to such awkward mechanics.

Done correctly, squats significantly enhance a workout, adding power and strength due to the size of the muscles being trained. Men can start with the Olympic bar, which weighs forty-five pounds. Women can start with the smaller straight bar, which weighs thirty pounds. The bar rests across your shoulders, your hands hold the bar, and your elbows are bent at an acute angle (Figure 6.17). Bend your knees until your thighs are parallel to the floor (Figure 6.18). Come back up by pressing your thighs and calves into the floor, rather than hauling yourself up by using your lower back muscles. Start with two sets of eight repetitions, building to three sets of twelve.

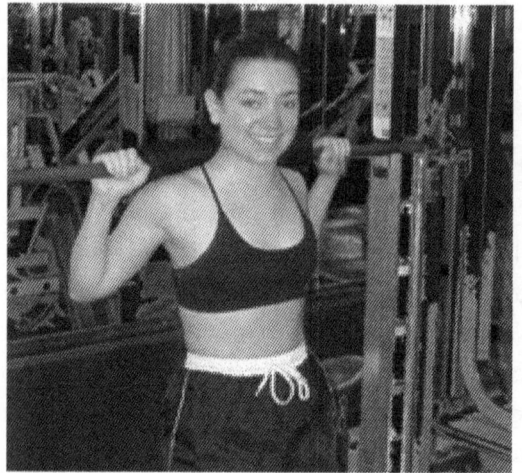 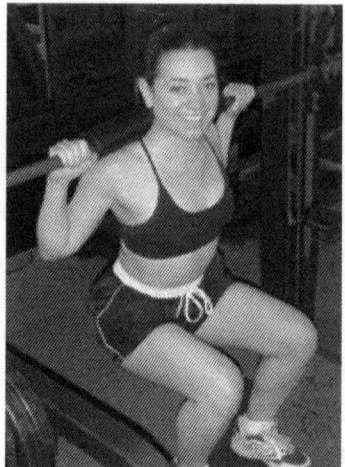

Figure 6.17   **Figure 6.18**

The quadriceps are trained in isolation by using the leg extension machine. This exercise is done in a sitting position. Adjust the seat so there is a slight bend to your knees when your feet are hooked behind the rollers (Figure 6.19). Straighten your knees in one smooth motion (Figure 6.20) and bend them again. Be sure to use equal energy in both legs, rather than emphasizing the power in one leg. Men can start with two plates (twenty pounds); women can start with one plate (ten pounds). Be sure that your thigh muscles are facing the ceiling during the exercise, rather than turning in or out. The image is to reach the thigh energy out through the calves and feet. Start with two sets of eight repetitions and build to three sets of twelve.

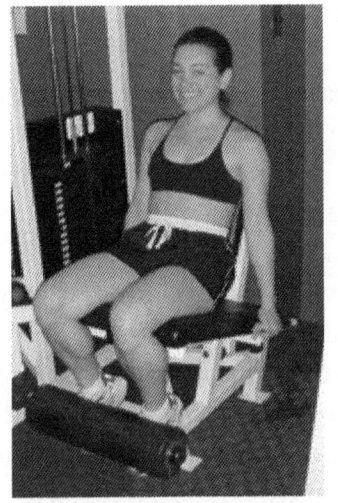
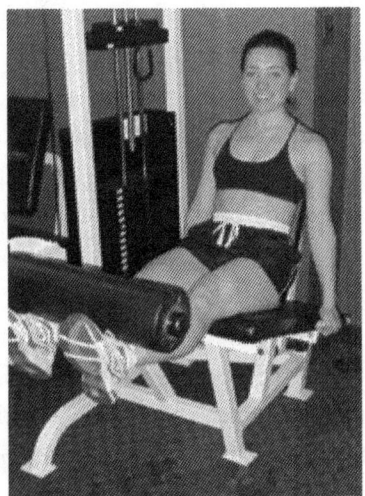

Figure 6.19   **Figure 6.20**

Hamstring curls are done lying on your stomach, utilizing a hamstring curl machine. This is frequently a bench with an obliquely angled bend—your abdomen is placed over that bend and your ankles hook under the foot rollers. Bend your knees, bringing the rollers toward your buttocks. This exercise trains your hamstrings, buttocks, and lower back muscles. Be sure to keep both hips on the bench; don't raise one side up to help move the weight. Don't arch the lower back to move the weight. The curl is a smooth steady motion. Start with two sets of eight repetitions and build to three sets of twelve.

There are two calf exercises: both use simple machines. One is done standing (this is for the gastrocnemius, the surface calf muscle) and one is done sitting (the seated exercise trains the soleus, the deeper calf muscle). In the standing toe raise exercise you stand with your shoulders snugly placed under two shoulder supports. Rise up onto the balls of your feet and return to a neutral position. A good beginning weight for a man might be six plates (sixty pounds). A good starting weight for a woman might be four plates (forty pounds). Start with two sets of eight repetitions and build to three sets of twelve.

Well-equipped gyms will probably have a seated-toe-raise machine. Sit with your knees bent, snugly placed under the padded support. Lift the support by rising onto the balls of your feet; then return to a neutral position. Men could start with twenty pounds; women could start with ten pounds. Do two sets of eight repetitions and build to three sets of twelve.

In general, it's time to increase the weight you're lifting when you can do three sets of twelve repetitions comfortably. How much do you add? Approximately ten percent. Sometimes it's a little more than ten percent, sometimes a little less. If you're working with dumbbells, go to the next heavier pair of dumbbells. For example, if you're doing biceps curls with ten-pound dumbbells, move up to the twelve-pounders. If you're working with fifteen-pounders, the next heaviest pair is usually the twenty-pounders (some well-equipped gyms have eighteen-pound dumbbells). If you can do bench presses with ninety pounds for three sets of twelve, use one hundred pounds the next time. Naturally, when you increase the weight the repetitions will initially decrease. Go back to three sets of eight and build up to three sets of twelve; then begin a new sequence of adding weight and decreasing repetitions.

I've just described a highly effective method of weight-training: start with three sets of six or eight repetitions at a manageable weight, and build to three sets of twelve repetitions at that weight. Then increase the weight by approximately ten percent, decrease the repetitions to three sets of eight, and build back up to three sets of twelve reps. Here's a review of our basic exercises:

- Bench press
- Lat pulldown
- Seated dumbbell press
- Biceps curl
- Triceps pressdown

- Squat
- Lower back extensions
- Abdominal training
- Quad extension
- Hamstring curl
- Standing toe raise
- Seated toe raise

This basic routine, not including the leg exercises (which are done on a separate day), will take about an hour. An hour is a good amount of time to be in the gym.

The variables of weight-training are types of exercise, amount of weight, and numbers of sets and repetitions. These variables can be combined in many different ways, each method leading to a slightly or dramatically different result. I'll describe a few combinations which are practical and effective, and relevant to any level of weight-training experience and skill.

We've discussed a primary approach of doing three sets of eight to twelve repetitions at manageable weights, and building sequentially. Once the weight becomes more substantial, for example, bench pressing one hundred twenty pounds, or doing biceps curls with thirty-pound dumb-bells, it may be more appropriate to do sets that lead up to that maximum weight. When I started weight-training, in my early thirties, after six months I could go to the gym, warm up, lay down on a bench, and do three sets of ten or twelve reps with one hundred fifty-five or one hundred sixty pounds. Now I do warm-up sets, building to one set of ten or twelve at my maximum weight.

Warm-up sets look like this. Let's say your top weight is eighty-five pounds for the bench press. Your first set of twelve reps would be at sixty-five pounds, the next set would be at seventy-five pounds, and your final set would be at eighty-five pounds. When you can do twelve reps at all three weights, start with seventy pounds the next time you do bench presses. Do a set of at least eight reps at seventy, then do a set at eighty, and do a final set at ninety pounds. When you can do twelve reps at each weight, move up to a beginning set of seventy-five pounds.

If your maximum lat pulldowns are at seventy pounds (seven plates), do a beginning set at sixty pounds, place a five-pound slug on the stack and do the next set at sixty-five pounds, and do a final set at seventy. When you can do twelve reps at all three weights, start your next lat session at sixty-five pounds, do the next set at seventy, and do a final set at seventy-five pounds.

This is a safe, highly efficient weight-training method. Here's a third approach to sets and reps: it's called "10-8-6-4-2". Do ten reps at a light weight, then eight reps at a slightly higher weight, and continue to add weight and reduce reps until you do two reps at a heavy, maximum weight. The bench press provides a good example. If your maximum bench press is one hundred pounds, start with ten reps at sixty-five pounds. Then do eight reps at seventy-five, six reps at eighty-five, four reps at ninety-five, and two reps at one hundred five pounds. You've just increased the maximum weight you can lift! Or, let's say you're a woman who has worked out for six months and can now squat one hundred pounds for eight reps. Use the same 10-8-6-4-2 approach and finish with two reps at one hundred five pounds. Or, you're a woman who does biceps curls with twenty-pounds dumbbells. Do ten reps at ten pounds, eight at twelve, six at fifteen, four at twenty, and do two reps at twenty-five pounds. You've increased your top weight!

We now have a series of basic exercises and some variety in our performance of these exercises, that is, the sets and repetitions. I know I need to vary my training routines or I get bored. There is a physiologic component to this restlessness. The kinesiologic structures (bones, muscles, tendons, and ligaments) are remarkably adaptive, and once these tissues have adapted their ability to make training gains is diminished. So, periodically varying your routine is useful both for your mental approach to exercise and the physiologic benefits of that exercise.

Fortunately, there are many ways in which we can vary our weight-training routines. The most basic method, of course, is to vary the specific exercises themselves. Let's add several exercises to our basic routines for each major muscle group.

The bench press is the basic exercise for the chest: it primarily trains the pectoralis major and is done lying flat on the bench. Another exercise for the chest is the incline bench press, done at an incline of approximately thirty degrees from the horizontal. The incline bench press targets the upper third of the pectoral mass; typically you can incline bench press about two-thirds of the weight that you can bench press. Press the bar straight up in the air. There is a tendency to lift the weight somewhat in front of your vertical plane: avoid this and lift the weight straight up.

A third chest exercise is the dumbbell flye. Flyes can be done lying flat or on an incline bench. Flat flyes are the basic version and train the bulk of the pectorals. Lie on a bench with your heels up on the bench at the end of the bench (this flattens out the lower back and provides good lumbar support). Variously, flyes may be done on an incline bench. Hold the two dumbbells overhead with a slight elbow bend (Figure 6.21). Your elbows are turned completely outward (the long axis of the dumbbells is in line with the long axis of the bench). Maintaining that slightly bent, turned outward elbow position, lower the dumbbells to the side: this movement opens the arms in a rough ellipse (Figure 6.22).

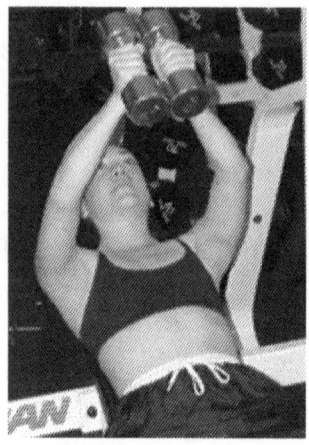

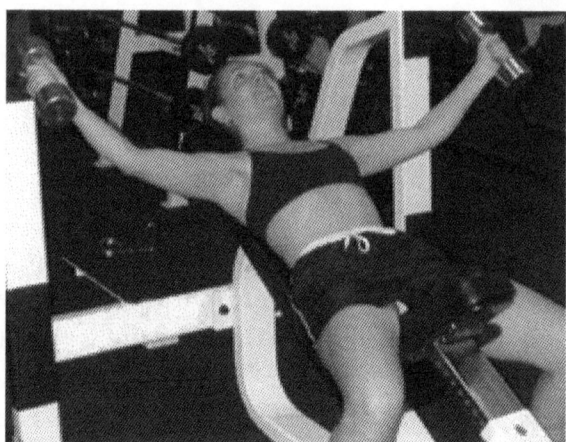

Figure 6.21   **Figure 6.22**

The dumbbells are lowered to a position where your elbows are in line with the sides of your body. Lowering any further than this may strain the pectoralis tendons. Utilizing the same elliptical movement, return the dumbbells to the upright position. If you're familiar with ballet, you'll recognize this opening flye movement as similar to the first *port-de-bras*. Incline flyes are similar; again, you'll use fifty to sixty-five percent of the weight used in flat flyes.

Two additional back exercises are the one-arm dumbbell row and the seated row. Let's start with the one-arm dumbbell row, using the right arm. We'll work on one of the portable flat benches. The weight is held in your right hand and you are standing on the right leg. The left side of your body is supported by the bench: your straight left arm supports your body in front and your left calf lies on the back part of the bench (your left front ankle is hooked onto the edge of the bench). Your right knee is bent about forty-five degrees and the weight is suspended straight down from your right shoulder (Figure 6.23). Your back is relatively flat. Lift the dumbbell in a rowing motion and aim the dumbbell toward your right hip (rather than lifting it up toward the middle of your back; Figure 6.24). Lower the weight. Women can probably start with ten-pound dumbbells; men can probably start with twenty-pounders.

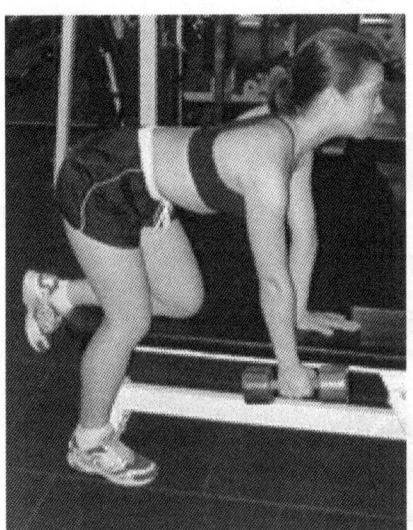 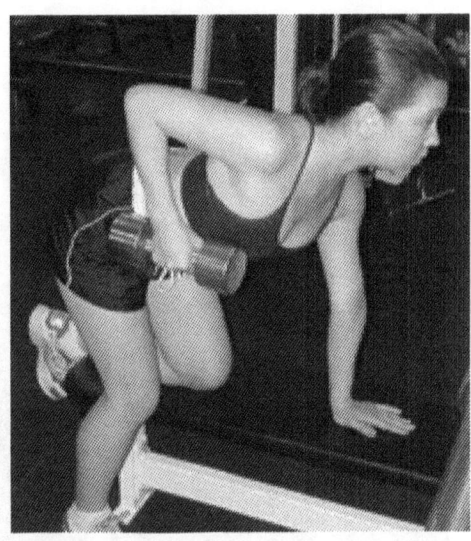

Figure 6.23   **Figure 6.24**

Seated rows are done with a rowing machine. Extend your arms to grasp the handles and bring your elbows back toward your waist in a rowing motion. Women can start with two or three plates (twenty or thirty pounds); men can start with four or five plates. Remember to concentrate and visualize the mass of the latissimus doing the work in both these back exercises.

A complete shoulder workout includes four exercises. We've already described the first one, the dumbbell or barbell overhead press. The shoulder overhead press is a compound exercise which trains the entire deltoid muscle. A useful principle is to start with a mass-building exercise like the bench press or shoulder press, adding other related exercises over time. Following the compound exercise for the shoulder, we'll train the anterior (front), middle, and posterior (rear) deltoid muscles.

Upright rows train the anterior deltoids. This exercise is done standing, with slightly bent knees. Grasp the center of the E-Z curl bar with both hands; your hands are about two inches apart and your arms are fully extended (Figure 6.25). Raise the bar to the level of your sternum (Figure 6.26) and lower it again.

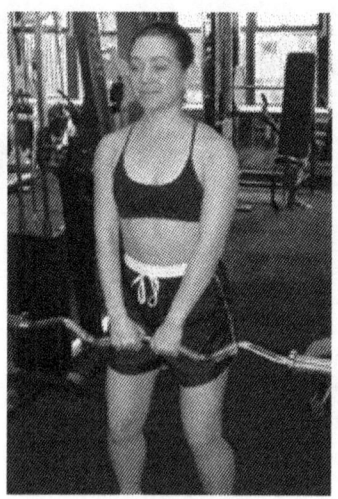
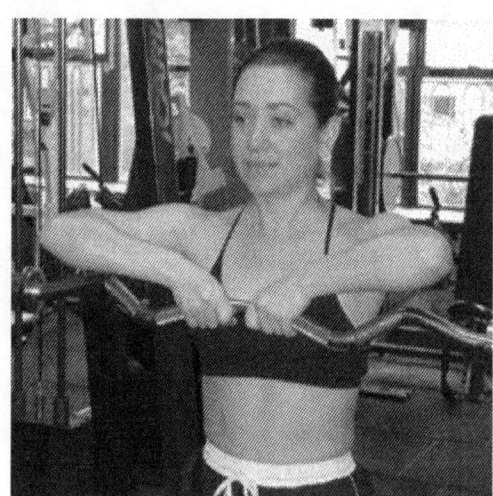

Figure 6.25   **Figure 6.26**

When you raise the bar your elbows bend, remaining parallel to the plane of your body. Be careful not to elevate your shoulders as you lift the bar—the shoulders continue to rest on the rib cage. Women can start with the bar itself (twenty pounds); men can start by adding five pound plates on either side (for a total of thirty pounds).

The middle deltoid is trained by the lateral raise. In a standing position, with slightly bent knees, hold two dumbbells in front of your pelvis so that your elbows are slightly bent and turned out (Figure 6.27). Raise both arms to just below shoulder height, maintaining a slight elbow bend (Figure 6.28), and lower the weights to the starting position.

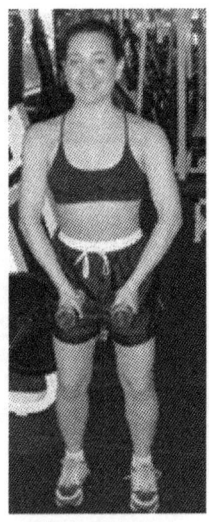
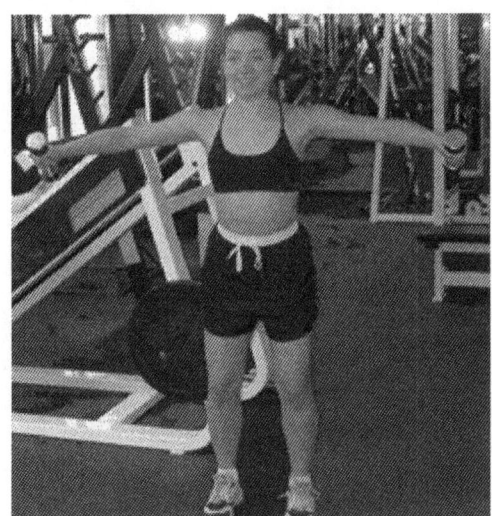

Figure 6.27   **Figure 6.28**

Be careful not to swing the weights; use muscle activity rather than momentum to move the dumbbells. Men can start with twelve-pound dumbbells; women can start with eight-pounders. An alternate lateral raise involves holding one dumbbell like a hammer, with the arm close to the side and the elbow bent at ninety degrees. Maintaining the ninety-degree elbow angle, raise your elbow ninety degrees to the side so that your elbow is at the level of your shoulder. Return the arm to the starting position. Do a set with one arm and then do a set with the other arm.

The posterior deltoid is trained by the bent-over row. Holding a dumbbell in each hand, sit on the edge of a bench and bend forward so that your chest is close to your knees and the dumbbells are close to the ground (Figure 6.29). Raise the dumbbells to the side to just below shoulder height (Figure 6.30), and then lower the dumbbells. This is a similar movement to the standing lateral raise, except that the prime mover is now the posterior deltoid. Women can start with three-pound dumbbells; men can start with eight-or ten-pounders.

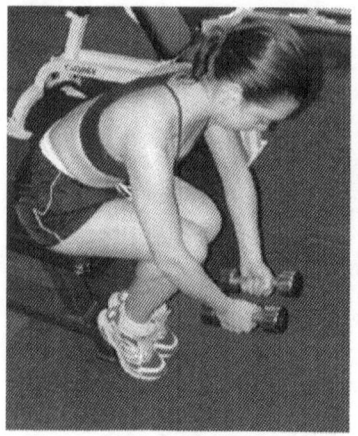
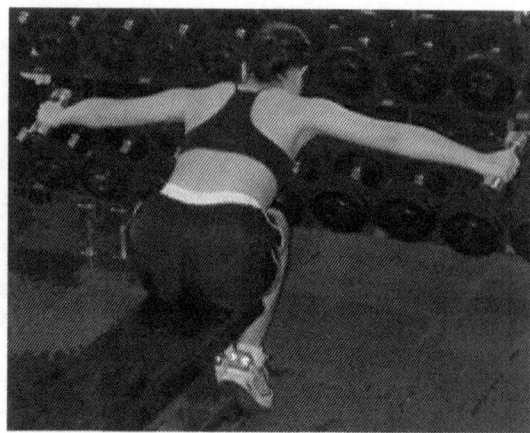

Figure 6.29   **Figure 6.30**

Additional biceps exercises include preacher curls and concentration curls. There is also an exercise called "21s". Preacher curls are done, naturally, on a preacher bench, which has a seat and a convex rectangular cushion which supports your extended arms. Preacher curls are best done with an E-Z curl bar; they may also be done with dumbbells. Place the E-Z curl bar on the supports, place your arms over the convex cushion, and grasp the bar in the middle with your hands about four inches apart (Figure 6.31). Curl the bar toward you as far as you can go, and then extend your arms fully (Figure 6.32). Preacher curls are an excellent biceps exercise. Men can start with five-pound plates on either side of the bar (thirty pounds total). Women can start with the bar itself (twenty pounds).

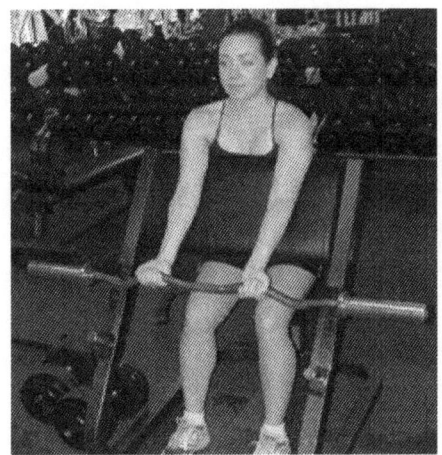

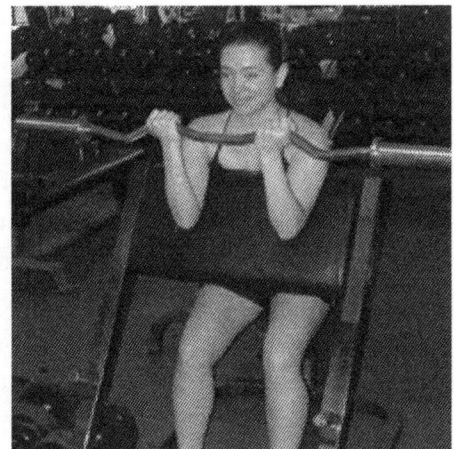

Figure 6.31   **Figure 6.32**

To do concentration curls with the right arm, sit at the end of a bench with your knees apart, hold a dumbbell in your right hand and let the dumbbell dangle inside your right calf. Place your left hand on the inside of your left knee for support, and then curl the right dumbbell upward, bracing your right elbow on the inside of your right knee. Do one set with your right arm. Then reverse the position and do a set with your left arm. Men can start with twelve- or fifteen-pound dumbbells. Women can start with five- or eight-pounders.

Here's an unusual and difficult biceps exercise: "21s". The exercise is done with the E-Z curl bar. 21s are done standing with the feet hip-width apart and the knees slightly bent. Hold the bar in front of you, at waist level, and curl the bar upward as in biceps curls (a movement of ninety degrees). Do this for seven repetitions. Then lower the bar all the way and curl the bar up to your waist (a movement of ninety degrees). Do this curl seven times. Then curl the bar from a fully extended position to a fully bent position. Do this last sequence seven times. Three sets of seven repetitions equals twenty-one! This challenging exercise will immediately pump up your biceps.

On to triceps extensions! Lying triceps extensions are done with an E-Z curl bar. Sit on the edge of a bench and grasp the E-Z curl bar with both hands in the middle of the bar: your hands are next to each other. Hold the bar close to you at about chest level. You then slide your hips about six inches toward the head end of the bench, and lie on the bench with your knees bent and your heels on the bench at the end of the bench. Now raise the weight off your chest so your arms are perpendicular to your torso, and bend your elbows so the bar is very close to your forehead. This is the beginning position (Figure 6.33). Using your triceps, extend your arms (straighten your elbows) so that your arms and forearms are in a straight line (Figure 6.34).

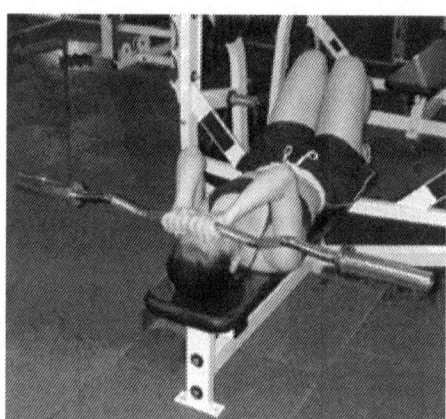
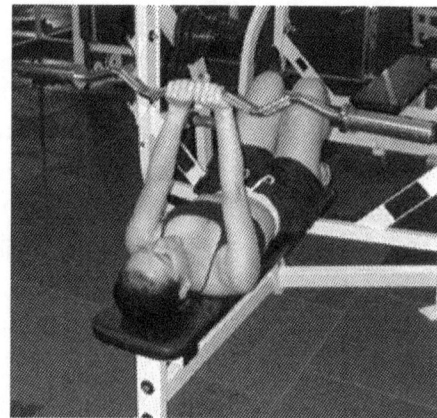

Figure 6.33   Figure 6.34

Then, maintaining your arms perpendicular to your torso, bend your elbows, lowering the weight back down to your forehead. This is one repetition. Women can start with the weight of the bar; men can start with an additional five or ten pounds (totaling twenty-five or thirty pounds). Be sure you are using your triceps for this exercise; it's easy to recruit your pectorals and perform this like a bench press. When you're doing lying triceps extensions correctly, you'll feel the weight immediately in the backs of your arms.

Triceps kickbacks are done utilizing the same setup as for one-arm rows (Figure 6.35). Let's start with the right arm. In this exercise you hold a dumbbell in your right hand with your elbow fully bent and close to your body. Supporting your body weight on your left calf and left hand, extend your right elbow fully (Figure 6.36). Your arm is now extended behind you. Return to the initial bent-elbow position. Do a set on the right and then a set on the left. Men can start with a ten- or twelve-pound dumbbell; women can start with a five- or eight-pounder.

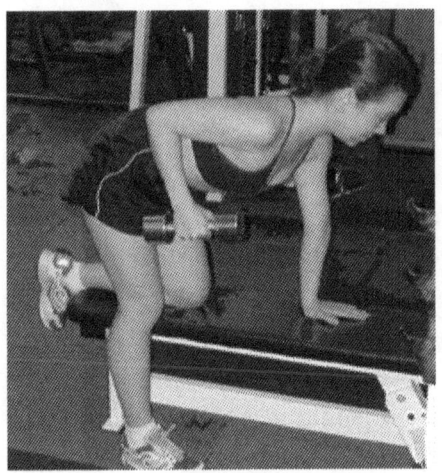 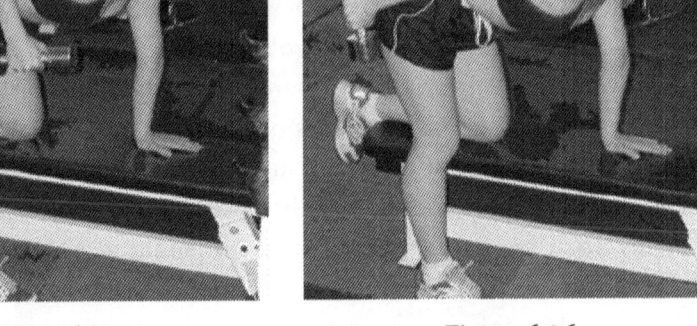

| Figure 6.35 | Figure 6.36 |

We now have at least three exercises for each of five upper body muscle groups: chest, back, shoulders, biceps, and triceps. We'll consider the biceps and triceps as one group, the arms, so we have four upper body groups in all. The lower body muscles, the quadriceps, hamstrings, and calves, will also be considered as one group: the legs. As you become more skilled in weight training, you will naturally get stronger and lift heavier weights. After about eight weeks of doing one exercise per muscle group, training all or most of the muscle groups each time you go to the gym, it's useful to start doing split routines. In split routines you only train two, or rarely three, muscle groups each session. The rest are trained the next time you go to the gym. For example, on Monday I could train chest and back; on Wednesday I could train shoulders and arms; and on Friday I would do legs. In a split routine system, each body part is trained heavily once per week.

Split routines allow you to work significantly harder. You only do two body parts per session (or one, if your split routine has legs on a separate day), but you do three exercises per body part, rather than the one exercise per group we had been doing as beginners. Exciting and gratifying strength gains become available, as well as rapid changes in muscle definition and body shape. Which split routine system to adopt? Remember, what works for me may not necessarily work for you. This principle is specifically applicable to split routines. You'll learn by experience the best combination for your body, but there are a few general guidelines.

I learned these principles the hard way. My first approach to split routines was to do chest and triceps on one day and back and biceps the next session. I had read about this routine in a weight-lifting magazine. It made sense: both the pectorals and the triceps are involved in pushing; the latissimus dorsi and biceps are involved in pulling. The routine worked well for about a year. However, I experienced a long run of training injuries once I began to lift what was for me heavy weight (about one hundred sixty-five for bench press and about one hundred thirty for lat pulldowns). I strained my pectoralis tendon, I strained my deltoid, I had various elbow injuries. I was discouraged and I was a mess. Each time I recovered from an injury and gradually returned to heavier weights, a new injury would occur.

I was talking this over with my friend Ben one day and he suggested I do a different split routine. He said the triceps are fatigued during bench presses and other exercises for the chest, and I was stressing them beyond their limits by doing three triceps exercises after three chest exercises. Similarly, the biceps are fatigued during back exercises. He recommended doing the large muscle groups on one day and the smaller muscles on another day. My new split routine was chest and back and then shoulders and arms. Alternatively, you could do chest and back one day, arms the next (since this is really two muscle groups, the biceps and triceps), and shoulders and legs on a third day. The back and chest—shoulders and arms split worked well. I exceeded my previous strength gains and never experienced the types of injuries as I did with my initial split routine.

Thus, a useful principle is to design a split routine that trains muscle groups that perform separate functions. Again, what works for some may not necessarily work for you. Experiment. Discover the training methods that are most effective for you. If you're *alive,* ready-to-go, and energized after a workout, then the system you're using is working. If you're sluggish, fatigued, and irritable after a workout, then you're overtraining and should consider altering your routine. You should always feel great after exercising. Being tired after exercising is not an appropriate physiologic response. You may need to drink water and eat because energy stores have been depleted, but any tiredness should be quite brief.

Another great benefit of split routines is that you are never doing the same thing two days in a row. Your kinesiologic system is forced to adapt, almost daily, to a new set of stimuli. Your soft-tissue structures are prevented from reaching a near-term homeostasis and continue to improve in strength and power. Also, from an intellectual perspective, you are continually engaged because the things you are doing are relatively different each day. Still, eventually you may become used to what you are doing, physically and mentally, and you plateau.

Varying your routines will keep everything fresh. Substitute a new exercise here and there. There are many exercises for each body part. Find a few new ones that work for you. Do an entirely different split routine, possibly back and shoulders one day, chest and legs another, and arms on the third day. Also, periodically, take some time off from lifting weights. A five- or seven-day rest from weight-training every few months will allow strength gains to be consolidated and provide necessary rest and recuperation. Within two weeks of your return to weight-training you'll notice an improvement in strength and endurance.

How long is a "good" workout? When you first start to do aerobic exercise, ten minutes is a good minimum and you build-up to a twenty-minute routine. Once you get going, thirty minutes is a useful standard for an effective workout. Plenty can get done in thirty minutes. And you can build to forty-five minutes or an hour of aerobic activity. When you start to lift weights, thirty minutes of work is a good beginning. A routine that includes one exercise each (three sets) for the five upper body groups, squats, lower back muscles, and abdominals will probably take an hour. An hour of lifting weights is a great workout. A split routine that includes shoulders and arms may take more than an hour, since you're doing nine different exercises (shoulders, triceps, and biceps).

The main point about time is that you should never be rushed. That's when the injuries happen. You're not thinking about what you're doing; you're thinking about where you're going to go and what you have to do when you get out of the gym. Your focus is elsewhere. Earlier we spoke about concentrating on the activity at hand and *seeing* the particular muscle group doing the work. When you're rushed this focus isn't possible. Lifting weights or doing any demanding physical activity requires specific attention. If your attention is not focused on the physical activity, you may get hurt. I'm aware this may sound naïve and idealistic. We're busy, it's a busy life, and sometimes it's barely possible to squeeze in a workout. I'm suggesting that once you have begun your training period, let that be your focus. Let your exercise be a form of meditation. Let it be a source of renewal.

By being present to the task at hand, whether running three miles or biking ten miles or doing a session with weights, you may locate a source of power that can be brought to the other responsibilities of that day. Training of yourself as an effective human being is an unlooked-for benefit of focused, intentional exercise. The *discipline* that is developed by engaging in a rigorous exercise program is naturally transferred to all our other accountabilities. One of the biggest thrills of exercising is setting training goals and ultimately exceeding them. This regular, consistent process of achievement provides a background of effectiveness for a person. You become used to doing the things you said you were going to do.

Accomplishment becomes a habit. Modest goals are set and achieved, ongoingly. I said I was going to run today and I did. I said I was going to do chest and back weight-training today and I did. I said I was going to stretch and ride my bike today and I did. I said that I would run a mile in eight-and-a-half minutes, and I did. I said I would bench press one hundred and fifty pounds and I did. This practice of manifesting your word in this way, saying you will do a thing and then doing it, provides benefit beyond measure in one's life.

Weight-training is an integral component of any exercise program. It may be the key element, supported by various aerobic activities, or it may be supplemental, providing cross-training for a person who is primarily a runner, swimmer, rollerblader, or bicyclist. Weight-training can be done by anyone of any age, with appropriate minor modifications. The physiologic benefits are extensive and long-lasting and the personal/human benefits are equally profound.

CHAPTER 7

▼

THE THREE "R"S: RUNNING, RATE, AND RHYTHM

I discovered running about ten years ago. I admit I had not understood running nor its benefits to that point. I had been on my junior high school track team, running sprints, but had not run as an adult. Having had various back problems, I didn't think I could run. In fact, my advice to patients with back pain was that they should not run. I had the hubris of many physicians and substituted the fact of my credentials for authentic facts based on direct experience. My professional license gave me license not only to practice but also to have an "expert opinion". Common sense suggested that the repeated concussive forces of running would be harmful for people with chronic back pain. I subscribed to this hypothesis; it was only when I started running myself that I experienced something completely different and quite unexpected. My back difficulties actually began to improve as soon as I began to run for exercise!

I don't intend this preamble to represent any sort of medical advice. There are individuals who will not benefit from running and for whom running may be harmful. There are several spine-related conditions that are not conducive to running, including disc herniation with documented nerve root compression, severe degenerative arthritis, spinal stenosis (narrowing of the spinal canal) with leg pain and weakness, and symptomatic spondylolisthesis (a type of spinal fracture that has healed, but with forward slippage of the vertebral body). Also, people with various inflammatory disorders, including rheumatoid arthritis and gout, will find that running is detrimental or, in fact, impossible. However, most individuals with chronic back pain do not have one of these disorders and can probably run, gaining great benefit and deriving tremendous satisfaction from doing so.

How do you know if you can run successfully? Start running. Slowly. As I mentioned when we were discussing weight-training, starting slowly allows you to make a real beginning. In running, if you do too much too soon, you will certainly aggravate a back problem or develop some other training-halting trouble such as shin splints or a hamstring strain. There really is no place for ego in exercise. Of course, I speak from bitter experience, having caused various foolish injuries by being, simply, foolish. So begin running gradually, slowly, and you will build incrementally to faster, longer runs.

Start by slowly jogging for ten minutes. That's enough for day one, even if you feel completely fine and want to do more. If you feel well the next day, that is, no problems have arisen, lightly jog for twelve minutes. Twelve minutes is very good for day two. Now, intend to run three or four times per week. From this point forward, you can increase your run by a minute a day until you're up to thirty minutes of running—fifteen minutes out and fifteen minutes back. If you are slowly jogging, doing about twelve minutes per mile, thirty minutes represents two-and-a-half miles. This is good. At this point, don't increase the duration of your runs; rather, increase your rate little by little. Run slightly faster for a portion of your run than you did the last time. Run slightly faster for a longer portion, or for a few portions, of your run than you did the last time. Lay out a track for yourself, using your car or a bike with an odometer. Measure a three-mile course. Measure a four-mile course. Over weeks, build up to running the three-mile course in thirty minutes: now you're running ten-minute miles.

Remember to improve speed gradually. I am very familiar with the need to achieve training goals *now*. However, this will not serve you. You may be able to meet that goal, today, by pushing, but there will likely be a price to pay in terms of recovery. For example, your legs may remain "heavy" for days and your next attempted run will be sluggish. You may be profoundly tired. Remember, strenuous exercise provides energy and enthusiasm for a person. If you feel *tired* for a few days after a particular training session, you'll know you did too much too soon. I don't want to be boring, but steady, incremental progress is best.

OK. You're running ten-minute miles for thirty minutes. Now you can begin to improve endurance—the amount of time you are running—and speed—how quickly you are running. Of course, speed is a synonym for velocity, that is, distance traveled per unit time (for example, one mile in ten minutes). Another variable is the combination of speed and endurance, that is, how fast you are running for how long. We'll look at each component of an effective running program. Right now let's discuss the physiologic benefits of running.

Everyone knows the major physiologic response to aerobic activity is improved efficiency of the cardiovascular system. This includes the heart, major arteries, arterioles, capillaries, venules, and major veins. The heart is an indefatigable pump that is powered by a neuroelectrical system. It is composed of specialized smooth muscle called cardiac muscle. It has been proposed that the heart is built to last one hundred and fifty years. Logically, if the heart beats less frequently per unit time it will last longer.

A given amount of blood needs to be received by the body's tissues per unit time (of course, this quantity varies with activity). If the amount of blood pumped with each heartbeat (or stroke) can be increased, the number of beats per minute will decrease. The quantity of blood pumped is called the stroke volume. One major effect of cardiovascular (aerobic) exercise is increased stroke volume: more blood is pumped each beat. The heart becomes more efficient, stronger, better able to manage bigger loads. The demands placed on the heart by vigorous exercise, particularly vigorous aerobic exercise, train the heart and make it a more efficient machine.

Blood supplies oxygen and other nutrients to the tissues of the body, including muscle. During aerobic activity muscle energy is provided by the metabolic breakdown of glycogen, which requires oxygen. The heart rate will increase to meet the increased oxygen demands, and as the heart trains, it becomes more efficient at pumping blood. So, over time you supply less energy to make the heart work; this saved energy can be applied to any other physical function. One useful method for evaluating stroke volume, or heart-rate efficiency, is to measure the resting pulse. The best time to do this is late at night, when you are truly resting. Aerobic exercise drives down the resting pulse; interval training (a specific type of aerobic exercise) reduces the resting pulse dramatically. For most of us, a resting pulse of 60 beats per minute is excellent. Individuals who don't exercise aerobically have resting pulses of 70 or more. These hearts are working twenty percent harder to supply the basic oxygen requirements of the body. Simply and bluntly, this is wasted energy—the machinery is in overdrive when it should be idling.

Another manifestation of cardiac efficiency is the reduced time it takes the heart to return to its baseline level. In other words, you've exercised hard and your heart rate is up. How long does it take your heart to return to a relative resting rate after the exercise is completed? Efficient hearts return to a slower rate in less time than do untrained hearts. This is not something you can easily quantify (there's no need to become an obsessive pulse-taker), but the benefits of this performance efficiency can be easily understood.

The rest of the cardiovascular system also benefits from aerobic exercise. Arteries and arterioles (small arteries) are lined by smooth muscle which contracts to circulate the blood. This smooth muscle undergoes a similar training effect and becomes more efficient, moving more blood per unit contraction. Importantly, the amount of pressure in the arterial system needed to circulate the blood can decrease as a result of increased muscular efficiency.

Thus, there are many profound, critically important physiologic benefits of aerobic exercise. Are they enough to get you out of bed in the morning, into your running shoes, and heading out the door? Possibly. There is also a noticeable feel-good response to running, based on endorphin production. We've heard of the "runner's high", popularized by the media during the running boom of the 1970s. This euphoric state is induced by increased levels of circulating endorphins, a naturally occurring opiate. Endorphins are distributed throughout the nervous system and are similar in structure to opium (derived from the poppy). They have several physiologic functions, including pain inhibition. Large concentrations make you feel *very* good. I would describe my own experience as variously tranquil, invigorated, satisfied, creative, harmonious, and centered. Quite a lot of well-being from a simple 45-minute run!

Running is one of the *key* exercises. If you can run, run. Running turns your body into a beautiful machine, creating long, sinuous muscular lines. Running basically trains everything: your legs, abdomen, spinal postural muscles, even your arms. It's funny about the arms. We don't think they are doing anything during running; the legs are doing all the work. But the arms are working too, pumping back and forth, or just maintaining a tonic, supporting, bent-arm posture. Even this tonic, steady position is work. The clearest evidence of the arm training effect is the increased arm strength available the next time you lift weights. Those extra couple of repetitions you didn't have the last time are a result of the four miles you ran the day before. And, of course, there is the cardiovascular benefit. The only training element running does not provide is a substantial strength and mass-building effect. Those things come from weight-training. So, naturally, the combination of running and weight-training provides a complete, powerful program. As I said earlier, I couldn't conceive how great running was until I started doing it.

Let's look at endurance first, and then we'll consider speed in the context of *interval workouts*. Endurance is how long you can keep going. I remember doing six-hundred-yard runs as a senior in high school and feeling pretty crummy afterward. My junior-high track days were three years behind me and my aerobic conditioning was gone. There was no way I could go out and run six hundred yards and feel good about it. Similarly, an adult can't start his running routine with a five-kilometer road race. Even fifteen minutes may be too much for the first few runs. As I noted earlier, start with ten minutes the first day. Build from there and your development of running fitness will be smooth and steady.

Where do you top out? That depends on your goals. If your goal is aerobic fitness, running between twelve and fifteen miles per week is perfect. This would translate to three or four four-mile runs per week or three four- to five-mile runs per week. More miles are not necessarily better. In fact, if you're not a competitive runner nor in training for half-marathons or marathons, running consistently more than fifteen or so miles per week is inappropriate and ultimately detrimental. Consistently running more than fifteen miles per week increases the likelihood of sustaining training injuries. Random injuries may occur to anyone; stuff *does* happen. However, it doesn't make sense to increase the risk of injury by inappropriate training. In the case of running, maximum aerobic benefit is obtained in the fifteen miles-per-week range. Additional mileage tends to improve aerobic fitness only marginally, while significantly increasing the likelihood of injury. Again, an ideal training regime would consist of three running days and two weight-training days per week.

Once you're at your average maximum workout mileage (three-and-a-half to five miles), you can begin to consider entering road races and, ultimately, increasing your speed. The best system for obtaining speed increases, for getting faster, is *interval training*. In interval training you run fast for a defined distance or time and then jog slowly for the same defined distance or time. *Running fast* means running slightly faster than your current race pace, utilizing a typical five-kilometer race time as your first benchmark. Running fast does not mean running full out. This misinterpretation of interval training results in profound fatigue, various thigh, calf, ankle, and foot injuries, speed *losses,* and elimination of interval training as part of one's routine.

One caveat about interval training. There is some arithmetic involved, because you are calculating interval times. It's easy, though, and you will get the idea of it quickly. Also, there's one additional piece of equipment that's needed: a runner's stopwatch. There are several brands available; the watch should include a setting for total elapsed time and another setting for a timer. The timer can be set to run down and stop, or run down and repeat.

OK. Let's say your 5-K race time is currently thirty minutes. That averages to approximately ten minutes per mile. Ten minutes per mile equals four 2.5-minute quarter-miles. If you're going to start interval training by running six quarter-miles, you will run these slightly faster than your race pace of 2 minutes and 30 seconds (2:30) per quarter. You will run these interval quarters at 2:25.

Before you go out, set your watch's timer for your interval time. Begin any interval session by lightly jogging for a mile or so. I do my intervals at the Central Park Reservoir. The distance from my apartment to the reservoir is 1.4 miles, so this distance serves as my warmup. To begin, do your first quarter in the designated time (2:25 in this example). Next, lightly jog a quarter-mile as a rest period. Next, run a second quarter at 2:25. Then lightly jog another quarter mile as a rest period. Do six quarter-mile sets in total, each set consisting of a fast quarter-mile and a slowly jogging quarter-mile. Including your mile or so of warmup, you've run a total of four miles. That's a great beginning. You will notice a speed increase almost immediately, even after the first interval workout. Also, you will notice you are passing a few more people, and it is slightly easier to run the hills on your route.

One interval session per week is recommended. One of the exciting aspects of interval training is the endless variety of combinations that can be done. First, the distances can be varied. One session might include six quarter-miles. You would build up to eight or ten quarters and then begin varying the lengths of the sets. Do a quarter-mile set (run fast, then lightly jog that distance), do a half-mile set, then another quarter and another half. This is the same total distance as six quarter-mile sets. The half-mile would be run slightly faster than your time for two quarters. If you're running 2:25 quarters, run the half-mile in 4:45 (this would be a 9:30 mile).

Another routine would be to run four half-mile sets. Another combination is the "stairstep": quarter-mile set, half-mile, three-quarters, one mile. In terms of distance, this is the equivalent of ten quarter-mile sets, or five total miles. If your quarter-mile is done in 2:25, do the half-mile in 4:50, the three-quarter mile in 7:15, and the mile in 9:45. If you're already running nine-minute miles (2:15 quarters), do quarter-miles in 2:10, half-miles in 4:20, three-quarters in 6:35, and one mile in 8:45. You can sense what this training will do to your race times!

Another variable in interval training is the manner in which you do the rest periods. In my rest periods I slowly jog the same distance that I ran fast. To do more overall work, you could slowly jog for the same *time* that you ran fast. If I am running 2:05 quarters, I would follow a fast quarter-mile by slowly jogging for 2:05. This would reduce the length of the rest period and increase the level of difficulty for the next repeat. This method is useful when you are running three-quarter-mile and mile repeats.

Bring your interval times down gradually. Knocking a single second off your quarter-mile repeats reduces your mile time by four seconds. It's easy to go too fast. I am continually resisting this temptation. The joy of running fast is so great and the sense of accomplishment so strong that I pull myself along, beating the chirping of the stopwatch by several seconds in many of my quarters. Now, although the space-time continuum will not break apart because you ran a quarter-mile repeat several seconds too fast, it's more efficient to run your intervals at the predetermined pace. If you ran too fast for much of your session, you may be fairly fatigued for a few days. That's how you know you overdid it. Also, during the interval session itself, if your times are slowing down in the last few repeats, you have been running too fast. Run your intervals just slightly faster than your race pace.

I remember the first 5-K race I ran after weeks of consistent interval training. Many New York City races are run in Central Park where the park drive itself is a ten-kilometer loop. Road races of five kilometers, four miles, and five miles are easily mapped out. The 5-Ks are run at the north end of the park where there is a series of *very* steep hills. Rollerbladers and bicyclists slow to a crawl on these hills. My friend Joe, a marathoner who has cerebral palsy, used to say, "I have great respect for the hills of Central Park". I huffed and puffed on those north-side hills during my first 5-K race. I thought, "When is this going to end?". There can be much pain and suffering on the north-end hills if you're not in good aerobic condition. I wasn't.

Remembering my first race, and having done some interval training, I set three goals for my next race: have enough reserve to be able to sprint the last minute or so of the race; be fast enough to pass some people (instead of always being passed); and do well on the north-end hills. I achieved all three! The best part was passing people on the *hills*. My aerobic fitness had increased dramatically as a result of my interval training. The payoff from intervals is almost immediate. Also, interval training drives your resting heartbeat *down*. When I'm doing intervals my resting pulse is in the forty-eight to fifty beats-per-minute range. This is a profound physiologic benefit.

Where will you do your interval training? You may live near a high school or college outdoor track, in which case you have a ready-made quarter-mile route. If not, you can lay out quarter- and half-mile routes using your bicycle's odometer. Map out a few, for variety. Running near wooded areas and running near the shore add a particular kind of beauty to your pursuit of fitness.

Both endurance and speed gains occur over time. It's a deep process. Of course, most of us want observable improvement: "How do I improve my race times? When will I be running faster?" Let's say you've run a 5-K race at a nine-minute-per-mile pace. You want to run miles in 8:45. This would be 2:10 quarters, approximately, and 4:20 half-miles, and 8:30 miles in interval training. Over a period of several months, gradually reduce your interval times to these levels and you will be running races at an 8:45 pace.

One of the great advantages of running is that it can be done anywhere. You are never limited by equipment and may only occasionally be limited by weather. Traveling? Just shove your running shoes, shorts, socks, and a few tops in your bag and you're set. Let's talk a little about equipment, and then we'll look at injuries and injury prevention.

The only equipment needed is running shoes. There are many companies making running shoes; these companies each make numerous models. How do you choose? You choose by following a few principles and using common sense. You know how in real estate only three things are important? (Location, location, location!). In running shoes, what's important is support, support, support! Good shoes have a stiff, yet flexible, sole. There is a stiff heel counter and antipronation cushioning. Your foot should be snugly supported by the shoe (the shoe shouldn't feel tight), and your big toe should be very near (not quite touching) the front of the shoe.

Good running shoes are generally ugly, with no hint of flash. Flashy style points generally indicate poor quality or poor product design. One company is generally acknowledged as the leader in running shoes. (Call your local running club to obtain its recommendations.) Make sure you can return the shoes for a full refund/exchange if they're not comfortable when you actually run in them. Most stores servicing runners will do this.

A good lifetime for a pair of running shoes is about one year. This represents about 750 miles (50 weeks times 15 miles per week). Buying a new pair each year will provide consistent protection and support for your feet, ankles, knees, hips, and lower back.

Let's look at some possible running injuries and their management. Please remember this is not an injury-prevention-and-treatment book; it's not a do-it-yourself sports medicine book. This is a how-to-have-a-body-that-works book, and in the context of running some comments on injury management are appropriate. Running injuries are almost all *overuse* injuries, and therein lies the method of injury prevention. Common overuse injuries include hamstring and calf strains, Achilles tendon strains, shin splints, metatarsal bruises, and metatarsal stress fractures. There are biomechanics-related pain syndromes including generalized knee pain and lower back pain. Acute injuries may occur as well, due mostly to circumstances. Stuff happens. (For example, you successfully locate that hidden tree root with the tip of your running shoe). Acute injuries include ankle sprains and bruises of various body parts (the ones that have struck the ground during a graceful (or graceless) fall.

We'll discuss overuse injuries first. Simply, if these injuries result from overuse, well, don't do that! As we noted earlier, if you are neither a competitive runner nor training for a long-distance race, fifteen miles per week is a good maximum. Doing more than that will predispose your bones and soft tissues to an overuse injury, each of which requires about six to eight weeks of rest and recovery. It's just not worth it. If you're new to running, build up endurance slowly. Allow your bones to remodel along physiologic lines of stress, becoming stronger and more resilient. Allow your muscles to become longer, your tendons to become more limber. Engage in the *process* of training.

Some people, specifically those with ectomorphic body types, are more susceptible to training injuries. Ectomorphic bodies are lean and long. On average, these body types experience more musculoskeletal injuries than do mesomorphs (increased muscle mass) and endomorphs (more prominent abdomen and soft body parts). The key to prevention of overuse injuries is cross-training, that is, adding another mode or method of training that provides a different focus. Weight-training is an important method of cross-training. It builds muscle mass, strengthens tendons and ligaments, protects joints, and trains the musculoskeletal system to withstand extreme loads throughout a maximal range of motion. Weight-training is the perfect complement to running. It is an efficient means for preventing running overuse injuries.

If you do experience an overuse injury, it's appropriate to stop running until the injury heals. Some injuries can be "worked through"; in other words, you can keep doing that sport at a modified level. However, the nature of an overuse injury necessitates cessation of the causative activity. Overuse injury represents tissue *failure:* failure of bone, muscle, ligament, or tendon. Here's a quick method of evaluating the seriousness of an injury, ordered in terms of increasing severity: (1) you only experience pain during the sporting activity; (2) you also experience pain during the activities of daily living (for example, walking); (3) you also experience pain during relative rest (for example, sitting or standing); (4) you also experience pain in bed. *Relative rest* is needed until the tissues are healed. Relative rest means that you avoid the aggravating activity but continue other types of training. If you're not running for six weeks or so, you may swim or ride a stationary bike (possibly), and certainly do weight-training for your upper body. Each of these will provide a good cross-training effect for your legs; you may even ultimately come back *stronger.*

Not a whole lot can be done about the "stuff happens" category. I was visiting the Outer Banks on the North Carolina coast recently, and was happily running on one of the local "jogging trails". Suddenly, with no warning, I fell flat on my face, banging my hip, knee, and forehead into the dirt. I had tripped over one of those deadly hidden tree roots! All I could do was laugh, pick myself up, shake off the dirt, and continue running my route back to the inn. I had some pain for the next day or so, but I didn't mind. I fell down. Big deal. Now, you could fall and break a bone, so I was lucky in that sense. Still, I will continue to run those "jogging trails" when available.

My point is that you can't run with your head to the ground, looking out for every branch and twig and bump in the road. Just pay attention. There's also something to be said for physical conditioning as a means of avoiding injury during an accident like a fall. When you are fit you are simply better coordinated. Your reaction times are that much faster because your body is used to working synchronously at a high level of performance (weight-training, running, swimming, dancing). In two falls that I can recall, I noticed I was falling forward, instantly concluded I couldn't regain my balance, and rolled into a forward somersault immediately after hitting the ground, finishing in a seated position. I had bruises on my hands and knees each time, but I hadn't hit my head or landed heavily on my pelvis. Conditioning allowed me to coordinate the sequence of the fall.

I have an analogy for the relationship between conditioning and injury modification during accidents. I have observed in my practice of chiropractic that individuals who are physically fit *always* get better faster than do those who are out of shape. It's practically a direct relationship. If you are fit your musculoskeletal problem is going to resolve quickly compared to that in a similar person who does not exercise regularly or who is overweight. If you are fit and fall while running, or turn an ankle, there will be less consequence than for a person who is not in shape.

Let's look now at the biomechanical types of pain patterns associated with running. The two main patterns involve lower back pain and knee pain, usually in both knees. I mentioned earlier that running helps improve chronic back pain. Some people report an increase in back discomfort or new back pain after beginning running for exercise. There are a number of possible causes of this. One cause is not stretching before you run. If the hamstrings, quadriceps, and/or calves are tight, there will be biomechanical strain on the lower back. Running certainly places demands on the soft tissues (muscles, tendons, and ligaments) of the lower back—if there is restricted mobility due to leg muscle tightness, there may be back pain as a consequence. Another cause of back pain is doing too much too soon. Start slowly, doing no more than ten minutes of running the first day or two. Don't try to run fast for the first few weeks. Your body needs to adjust to the demands of running; inappropriate speed may result in strains and/or sprains.

A third cause of lower back pain is bad equipment. Your new running shoes don't fit properly, you didn't buy a pair that was sufficiently shock-absorbing, or you thought you could run in your tennis sneakers or "cross-training" shoes. You can't. "Cross-training" shoes are for weight-lifting and aerobic equipment such as stair machines, stationary bikes, and treadmills. Running requires running shoes. Your equipment is not the best place to save money. Bargain brands will not provide appropriate protection and support.

The fourth cause of lower back pain during running is stress. Stress is insidious, has profound and subtle physiologic consequences, and may be implicated in a wide variety of rheumatic, immunologic, and degenerative disorders. Interestingly, being aware of stress as a causative factor in lower back pain has brought it increasingly to my attention. This is not to suggest that the problem is in one's "head". The physiologic effects can be observed and the pain produced by the biomechanical dysfunction is real. In the context of running, stress shortens and tightens lower back muscles. With stress, these muscles are chronically contracted (here, *chronic* implies a pattern of holding a muscular contraction, possibly for as little as several hours). Even if you have stretched, stress reaction may reinitiate muscular tightening, causing lower back pain during running.

To recap, the large majority of people should be able to run relatively pain-free. Causes of back pain during running include failure to stretch, doing too much too soon, poor equipment, and stress. The first three can be corrected in a straightforward fashion, adding understanding and intentionality to the choice of running as an exercise. The removal of stress as a causative factor may require something more subtle, an inner awareness rather than external action. It's useful to identify stress as a cause of pain. Something *can* be done about it, you can enjoy the beautiful sport of running, and you can run pain-free.

Being able to run is a great accomplishment for people who have run before and sustained an injury which has prevented them from running. My two main goals as a chiropractic physician are to reduce and/or resolve a person's pain and return him or her to physical activity, since ultimately it is the physical activity, the exercise, that will keep a person well. A recent patient, a young woman named Lisa, came to see me for treatment of neck and lower back pain which resulted from a serious car crash. She was lucky, in a sense, having only sustained musculoligamentous injury. Lisa is a runner, but had not been able to run since the accident, which occurred about two months previously. She was feeling much better after two treatments, traveled for two weeks on business, and returned for her third visit looking quite well. Lisa proudly reported that she had started running and "felt great"! "You know,", she added, "my back loosens up when I run." Now, she had started running a *little* sooner than I would have recommended, but she was fine. Her objective findings were all reduced, and she was back in control of her schedule. Lisa could do what she wanted to do, what her body deeply needed to do—engage in strenuous exercise. She could run.

A few years ago I began treating a 35-year-old woman named Jessica for chronic neck and upper back pain. Jessica is a painter, an abstract expressionist, and supports herself as an administrative assistant. Her long-term physical ailments were wearing her down, taking a toll on her productivity as an artist. She had never exercised much and hadn't done any exercise at all for years. It wasn't part of her self-concept. Jessica is an artist; none of her friends exercise either. Her treatment progressed well; after about three months she was about fifty percent improved. She experienced less pain, less often, and her physical activities were less bothersome. At this point she plateaued and did not improve over the next month or so. All along, we had been talking about the usefulness of exercising, but Jessica had resisted putting this into her life. Exercise was foreign: it was something other people, those who weren't artists, did. Plateauing in treatment was the motivating factor: she wanted to get well and began to understand she could not merely be a passive participant.

Jessica began to run. She started slowly, as we have described, and increased her time and distance gradually. Now she does training runs of four or five miles, consistently. She runs road races! One day Jessica came to my office and asked, "What do you think about weight-lifting for me?" I answered that it would be beneficial, so she joined a gym and started to lift weights. It was an easy decision, since her self-image now included physical fitness.

Jessica is now an athlete as well as an artist and is unrecognizable to herself and her friends. Her body has altered dramatically. Jessica had minimal muscle tone when we first met; she wasn't overweight but was carrying extra padding in her abdomen, buttocks, and thighs. Her complexion was sallow and her posture rigid from tension and pain. Most of the fatty tissue is gone; her muscles are hard with good definition. She's had various minor training injuries, all fairly typical and all resolved on a short-term basis. We don't see each other much anymore, which is how I intend things to turn out. Help people get better, teach them to do things that will keep them well, and send them on their way.

Jessica is a good example of this treatment design. She has undergone a remarkable transformation through her exercise program. She loves her new body and her new life. Her experience is inspiring, but neither unusual nor unique. It is an expected outcome of a consistent, well-designed, enjoyable exercise regime, an experience that is available to everyone.

Running provides perceptible, and frequently outstanding, physiologic benefits. It does take something, however. Vanessa, a 42-year-old patient, asked me the other day, "When does it get easier? When does it take less effort?" I am familiar with this refrain. I live on York Avenue in Manhattan, the easternmost avenue on the Upper East Side. My runs begin by running to Central Park, whose eastern border is Fifth Avenue.

The initial portion of this York-to-Fifth run is uphill, all the way to Third Avenue. I don't get to start my runs with a nice, easy flat jog. My runs begin uphill. For the first few minutes, I often wonder, "Exactly why am I doing this?" It's painful to start these runs, it's slow, I don't like the huffing-and-puffing part, blah, blah, blah.

Only recently, after about four months of good consistency (I hadn't run much last winter), my initial uphill run has become easier. Now I just do it, without the experience of burden and difficulty. But it took that long to get there. Also, during a run I have various body sensations. At some points I feel powerful and free, at other points I slog along and my legs feel heavy. I expect the fatigued feeling will pass, however, and after a little while it does, and I am back to feeling strong and well.

At this stage of my running career, I am familiar with these transient sensations and don't pay much attention to them. I am out there running and doing what I said I was going to do. And I am well aware of the expansive, thrilling experience of well-being and accomplishment that is present at the conclusion of a run. I know what will be present at the end and I will put up with the work that running sometimes is to achieve that result.

Recently, I have been training myself to be present to what I'm doing while I'm doing it, training myself to enjoy and savor all the aspects and segments of my run. Rather than thinking about how great I'll feel at the end, or wishing I were at the downhill portion of my run, or how much time is left and should I make my run shorter today, I am working on experiencing my body working throughout my run. Yes, my body is working, it's working hard, as it was designed to do. I am experiencing my body as a machine, infinitely complex and brilliantly constructed. Each stride represents power, grace, beauty, and agility. If this is my focus, if I am present to the *machinery* and the *artistry,* there is no room for *effort* and *struggle,* no room for *tiredness* and *fatigue.* And I am now freer to run. Yes, the uphill parts are work and I may be breathing heavily. Yes, I may slow down, sometimes significantly, for some parts of my run. But this doesn't mean that I'm *tired!* My machinery is working appropriately for a specific task, and I am in *training*. If I continue training long enough, the difficulty of the various tasks of running will lessen and I will run more lightly and swiftly.

There *is* pain in running. I don't want to hide or gloss over this fact. Pain is a part of any repetitive physical activity, whether bike riding, swimming, or running. Pain is a part of most sports, whether football, soccer, basketball, or tennis. As a dancer, I was very familiar with pain. One of my jazz dance teachers, Fred, used to say, "Love the pain". Fred had the right idea. In sports and athletic activities such as dance, pain usually implies you have reached your current physical limit and are experiencing the physical pain of exceeding that limit. Or you got knocked around and are hurting. So what? Keep going. This is interesting. Loving the pain is a life-defining concept, *and* you need to be able to distinguish good pain from bad pain. Sometimes, pain means *stop*. How do you learn to differentiate good pain from bad pain?

First, it's important to acknowledge that it's OK to experience pain. This is what Fred meant. If you are new to exercise, physical pain may be quite unfamiliar and unpleasant; you may think you're doing something wrong or are hurting yourself. You're probably not. The demand of muscles for oxygen, the accumulation of metabolic end-products such as lactic acid, the stretch of tendons and movement of joints beyond their accustomed limits, all of these create temporary pain. These things are fine and physiologic. In football, dance, gymnastics, and running, participants are continually testing their physical limitations. There will be pain. It's powerful for a person to consider pain as simply a reflection of hard work. Pain is a signal from the machinery, an indicator light on the flight console.

What about the pain that is "bad" pain, the pain that means you have sustained an injury and should stop your activity? "Good" pain is typically experienced as an achiness or soreness; there might be a sharp sensation, but it's transitory and does not return. Sharp pain that persists means *stop*. Burning pain means stop. Significant soreness that *really* hurts means stop.

Certainly, swelling of a joint means stop. Of course, these comments are quite general. You will develop a sense of what's happening in your body and become skillful at distinguishing normal exercise discomfort from the pain of injury. My point is that many of us, as adults, are rather removed from consistent patterns of exercise. Initiating an exercise program will produce physical discomfort, even some pain, and this is all OK. Slow, progressive adaptation will eliminate most of the sports-type injuries that bring people to my office for treatment. I first heard Fred's love-the-pain dictum almost thirty years ago, in Amsterdam in the summer of 1972. This principle has provided a great sense of freedom. I can have a body that works.

I've begun to experience something unusual on the other side of the work of exercise: I now am *gliding* through my workouts. Running and lifting weights are not particularly easier, but there is less effort involved. There is less work. I have concluded this *gliding* is a result of consistency, and possibly a benefit of combining running and weight-lifting. It might be a physical result, but it's a new experience for me.

For example, a recent interval workout consisted of eight quarter-miles at 2:10, a good intermediate speed for me. There was a long gap until my next interval session, a four-week hiatus. I thought I would run 2:10 quarters again, since it had been four weeks. My first quarter-mile was 2:05, not really a surprise since the first quarter is usually faster than I intend it to be. However, I ran each successive quarter-mile in the same 2:05, and it was pretty *easy.* I could have run faster, knew I shouldn't because I was already running relatively fast, and had a breakthrough session. Usually the last quarter-mile is slower because I have worked hard and pushed myself. This last quarter was not like that: it was the same 2:05. When I was finished I felt like I hadn't done very much at all. I *glided* through that workout.

There has been a subtle shift in my approach to exercise and my experience of the exercise sessions themselves. Also, I notice I have been taking on my running and weight-training as a self-expression. These activities are becoming an expression of who I am, rather than something I have to do or something that will get me to a particular place. I say: I am physically fit. I am healthy and well. Therefore, for me, exercise is a self-expression, it is an outward manifestation of my self-image.

And, there's another possibility: Can "gliding through my workouts" be transferred to the rest of my day, to my other accountabilities? Can I bring this new ease, this new grace, to my relationships, occupation, and family? I experience *gliding* as smooth and straightforward. There is effort but no struggle. The surface is glass, I have momentum, and I am sailing along. What would life be like if we lived it with such clarity, elegance, and style? I'd like to propose that this experience of graceful exercise, of being "in the zone", can make a profound difference in one's other pursuits in life, and can in fact be a wonderful metaphor for living well.

CHAPTER 8

▼

REAL NUTRITION FOR REAL PEOPLE: GUIDELINES FOR HEALTHY EATING

So much has been written about nutrition. There are books on how to lose weight and how to gain weight, and books on what to eat and what not to eat if you have this disease or that disorder. There are nutrition books for senior citizens, bodybuilders, and women who are pregnant. There is an enormous amount of excellent material available in any bookstore or library. One challenge is to make sense of it all, to learn some key concepts that are applicable to a wide range of situations. Another challenge is presented by the often contradictory nature of authoritative reports. The question of cholesterol and fats in general is representative of this kind of issue. First, fats were no good for you. In particular, cholesterol intake should be monitored closely. Then, there were "good" and "bad" cholesterols. Lately, there's been a lot of revision of the whole question of saturated versus unsaturated fats. For years, margarine was superior to butter. It now appears that margarine is "bad" and butter is OK, despite containing lots of saturated fat.

It certainly seems that nutritional concepts are in flux and that it's a confusing topic area. Most of us would like to have a reasonably healthy diet, but the framework for what constitutes "healthy" is not clear-cut. In this chapter we'll sort through some of the controversy, and provide sound dietary principles which can guide the vast majority of people to make choices that serve both their taste buds and their fitness goals. I'm going to simplify the entire nutritional process—not by "dumbing it down", but rather by emphasizing strategies that actually work.

Let's start by acknowledging that few people have time to prepare and cook complicated meals. People work late hours, have business or social engagements after work, or exercise before going home for the night. Frozen food, fast food, and take-out comprise much of our dinner eating. Breakfast is coffee and a bagel or muffin; lunch is a sandwich or burger or sometimes nothing. This is the busy reality, most of the time. Long lists of "good" foods to eat probably don't provide an effective solution, and indirectly create guilt that we're not eating the foods on the list. No one wants more guilt.

For most of our lives we've been bombarded by advertisements and magazine articles about the negative effects of certain foods and the beneficial effects of others. Each decade has its special "healthful" foods and "don't-eat-that!" foods. Red meat is good for you; red meat is bad for you. Milk is good for you; milk is bad for you. Tomatoes, onions, and green peppers are good for you; these vegetables are bad for you. Eat a serving of broccoli every day; eat a serving of bran every day; eat a serving of omega-3 unsaturated fish oils every day. Who is going to pay attention to all this and actually construct their diets like this? And, what happens to you when you've been following the current crest of advice about a particular food group and that crest suddenly turns into a trough?

In this sense, nutrition has been very much like fashion. Styles come, and they go. Shorter hemlines; longer hemlines. Two-button sport jackets; three-button sport jackets. Is following the nutritional fad of the moment the best we can do? Are isolated bits of information taken out of the larger context the best we can hope for? I propose that the bottom line on nutrition is common sense. Again, I don't intend to be simplistic. I do suggest that simple, basic principles exist, the implementation of which will lead to easy, healthy food plans—ones which can be followed without guilt!

Media discussions of size and weight are equally as common as material on which foods to eat. Americans tend to get overweight. Food is abundant and exercise, in general, is inconsistent. This combination will put weight on a person. Is the poundage the problem, though, or is it the lack of conditioning? The two are interconnected, of course, but I suggest that, overall, conditioning is the more critical factor. It's well known that dieting alone will not cause permanent weight reduction. You lose thirty pounds, and three months later you've gained thirty-five. Next year you lose twenty-five pounds, and six months later you've gained back thirty. The missing element is consistent exercise.

Here's a useful question: What is the optimal weight for a particular individual? This question is often not considered: You're a five-foot-five-inch woman, you should weigh 115 pounds. You're a six-foot tall man, you should weigh 175 pounds. This facile figuring does not account for variations in human form. Ectomorphic body types are naturally slender; mesomorphic types have more muscle bulk and are sturdier; endomorphic types are rounder, more abdomen-oriented, and more readily store fat. A six-feet tall male endomorph will naturally weigh more than an ecto-morph of equal height.

Let's say a good weight for such an endomorph is 210 pounds. If this 210-pounder tries to get down to 180 pounds to meet some prescribed weight-to-height ideal, he will experience a great deal of misery. He would have to consume drastically less calories, which would create other health issues. So, rather than describing weight-to-height relationships on a mono-valued basis (that is, if you are height *X,* you should be weight *Y*), we can more effectively use relative scales based on body type. In this system, a good weight for a six-feet tall ectomorph would be 170 or 175, a fit mesomorph would weigh about 190, and a fit endomorph would weigh about 210.

A 250-pound endomorph now has about forty pounds to lose to get to a good, healthy weight. This is doable and far more realistic than dropping seventy-five pounds to reach 175. This person will never reach the ectomorph's weight, will become unwell trying to get there, and may eventually drift back to the original overweight state. The conclusion? "It's too hard to lose weight, it never stays off anyway, so why bother? Why not just enjoy myself?"

Here's something else to think about regarding the readout on your digital scale. Weight should not only be considered in the context of body type, but also with reference to the overall muscle bulk/body fat relationship. Two things are implied here. First, someone who weighs an appropriate amount for his height (say, 170 pounds for a six-foot ectomorph) is not necessarily fit. Compare two 170-pounders. One is a runner, with strong legs and well-balanced upper body musculature. The other is sedentary, with a slightly stooped posture, a small paunch, and minimal muscle tone. One is clearly fit; the other is clearly not. Thus, weight alone is not a sufficient criterion for fitness. Consider a 220-pound mesomorph. We might think he needs to lose about twenty pounds to meet average weight standards. However, if those twenty pounds represent lean muscle mass, added over a period of several years of conditioning, then 220 pounds is an effective weight. Weight is relative. In order for a person's weight to be a useful measure of health, it should be evaluated in relationship to both body type and level of fitness.

Often, *losing weight* is not the issue; rather, conversion of body fat to lean muscle mass is the unrecognized goal. We've established that about 210 pounds is OK for a six-foot endomorph. Now, is this person fit or not? If he's an average American, he's not fit. He only meets the average standard for weight matched to body type. He starts a fitness program, thinking that one of the benefits will be weight loss. He wants to lose weight, he's been heavy all his life. Surprisingly, and to his possible annoyance, his weight stays constant for the next three months, even though he's exercising three times a week. He may even add a couple of pounds! What's happening here? What's happening is that fat stores are being reduced and muscle mass is increasing. Muscle weighs more than fat. Depending on the intensity of exercise and the average amount of calories consumed, such a person's weight will remain steady or even increase a little. Over time, with consistent exercise, the 210-pounder may not have lost much weight, but his level of conditioning will have improved dramatically. He might become an "endomorph/mesomorph", and his weight would be appropriate.

How do you know if your weight is a good weight? Trust your instincts on this—you know the answer to this question. If there are a lot of dairy products, sugar, cake, candy, cookies, bagels, olive oil, and sticky buns in your diet, you're overweight. If you eat ice cream every other day, you're overweight. If you haven't exercised in more than two months, you're over-weight. Is your belt comfortably closing at the second notch instead of the third? Is the dress you bought three months ago tighter around the waist? You're overweight.

You might say, "OK, I'm carrying a few extra pounds. What's the big deal?" Well, yes, on one hand, it might *not* be a big deal. I'm not suggest-ing everyone fit into standardized norms for height and weight. However, there are real health concerns associated with maintaining excess body weight over the long term. If we're interested in creating happy, fulfilled, creative, rich lives, then optimization of physical health, including weight management, becomes a related goal.

What are some of the problems associated with excess weight? Extra weight implies additional cells and tissues; these structures require a blood supply to provide oxygen and nutrients and remove metabolic waste. The cardiovascular system is burdened with additional work. Similarly, extra work is done by the pulmonary system in order to provide sufficient oxygen for an overburdened system. Fatty deposits may accumulate on the inner walls of blood vessels, narrowing their internal dimensions. This will create an ongoing rise in blood pressure to force blood through the narrowed openings. Excess weight stored as fat does not participate in the day-to-day management of body systems: it is simply just lugged around, creating additional work for the bones, joints, and muscles. And, more food is needed to provide energy for the overworked systems, stressing the resources of the systems manager—you!

The bottom line is simple physics: extra weight implies extra work. Extra work that doesn't produce anything useful is wasted effort; it's inefficient. Lean machines are efficient machines. Efficient machines need less maintenance, break down less often, and last longer. What we'd like to do here is increase the efficiency of your machine. This interpretation of weight reduction becomes possible if we can clear the emotional background usually associated with weight concerns.

It's important to emphasize that nothing is wrong. If one is overweight, one is overweight. If one is thin and out of shape, one is thin and out of shape. That's it. There's no judgment in such an evaluation, no "goodness" in being lean as opposed to anything else. If I can give up my evaluation of myself as "good", "bad", or whatever in relation to my weight, then I will be able to manage my weight. If not, my hidden issues will control events: I'll lose weight with one set of intentions, and put weight back on as a result of my undistinguished concerns and fears. Some self-investigation might be useful here, particularly with respect to two questions. The first question is, What am I getting out of being overweight? The second question is, Who do I think I'd have to be if I weighed less and was better conditioned? The answers to the first question are those factors keeping a person out of shape. The answers to the second question are those factors keeping a person from staying in shape. The answers are personal, individual, and probably *not* obvious. These questions represent an inquiry; they can be posed in relation to many of our issues and concerns. There are no "right" answers. The benefit is in the process of inquiring. Choose to have an efficient body weight, choose to become fit, and keep looking, observing, and inquiring.

What follows may appear to be a conversation on how to lose weight. It is really a discussion of how to be fit, that is, how to maintain optimal weight and health. So if you're already at a great weight, I believe this information will still be useful and valuable.

How to get there? How to get to where we want to go, that is, how to reach a target optimal weight? Let's start by setting realistic targets with realistic time frames. For example, losing fifty pounds (going from 260 to 210 for a six-foot male endomorph) might seem completely undoable. An impossible task. How will I ever lose fifty pounds? Forget that. Lose ten pounds. Then, having worked off ten pounds and reached 250, set the next target of ten more pounds. And so on, all the way down to 210. You can see that I'm not proposing a quick-weight-loss solution. Weight lost rapidly through a special diet or prescription will be put back on soon thereafter. The missing ingredient in quick-fix programs is the commitment to shift how one has been living. Effective weight loss occurs in the context of lifestyle modifications that address both healthy eating patterns and exercise. Here's the bad news: there is no magic solution for weight loss. The good news is that excess weight does not return when habits of healthy diet and exercise are maintained consistently.

The recommendation is to lose weight slowly, over time. This will take an ongoing commitment to fitness. What's a good recommendation for weight loss relative to time? Probably six or eight pounds a month. This is reasonable, doable, and doesn't involve torturing yourself. How do you lose weight? Well, once I acknowledge that I intend to lose weight and regain fitness, and also that I intend to lose weight responsibly and gradually, the steps to take are really pretty simple and straightforward: Drink water. Eat less. Manage the fat in my diet. Begin consistent aerobic exercise. That's it. No stimulants, no diuretics, no special drinks or preparations. Now, it takes something to be on this particular weight-loss program. It's a program of personal responsibility. Such a program will provide lasting benefit, flowing from the things I learn about myself along the way. OK. Let's lose some weight.

Drink water. The recommendation to drink more water is the most important nutritional advice anybody can give anybody else. If you're not drinking enough water, whatever else you're doing with respect to nutrition will have a diminished impact. If you're not drinking at least four glasses of water a day, your internal environment is toxic. I mean that, really. Toxic. About seventy percent of the human body is composed of water. Both the intercellular matrix that holds cells together and the intracellular matrix that supports the internal cellular organelles (such as ribosomes, mitochondria, and Golgi bodies) are largely composed of water. Blood is mostly water. Sufficient water is necessary to maintain a homeostatic biochemical environment, so that energy is obtained, stored, and utilized effectively. We burn energy twenty-four hours a day and produce various types of metabolic waste. Sufficient water is necessary to remove these waste products (such as lactic acid, an end-product of muscle metabolism). If metabolic end-products accumulate, internal "pollution" develops. Drinking more water will cause you to urinate more frequently, which of course is part of the process of waste removal.

How much water is enough to be healthy, that is, to maintain optimum physical functioning? Well, you can never drink too much water. Any excess is excreted. The problem, as we've described, is drinking too little. There are benchmarks suggesting that eight glasses a day are needed. My sense is that this number is too high for many people. Since most of us are barely drinking two glasses of water a day, drinking four or five glasses a day is realistic and doable. Speaking generally, sufficient water intake has a beneficial effect on digestion, respiration, metabolism, and excretion. Observable benefits include decreased incidence of upper respiratory infections, improved skin tone, and more restful sleep. With respect to weight loss, increased water intake is necessary in the context of aerobic exercise.

Eat less. I know, this is stating the obvious, but it really is a main point. If you are committed to losing weight over the long term, you will be committed to eating less. This is a definite lifestyle modification. You are storing excess food intake as fat because those nutrients represent an over-supply: you are consuming more food than is necessary to maintain daily functioning. There are two main solutions here: eat less and exercise more. A corollary solution involves modifying the amount of fat consumed each day. Thus, eating less is one of the requisites for losing weight. This does-n't mean starve yourself. Eating less involves putting less food on your plate, not eating additional portions, considerably reducing intake of breads and bagels containing processed flour, markedly reducing cake and candy, and not eating between meals (the exception might be to have a banana or an apple).

We'll talk later about meal construction, but for now let's think of meals as simply breakfast, lunch, and dinner. There will be initial discom-fort, stomach pangs or growling, as your gastrointestinal tract becomes accustomed to decreased stimulation. These sensations will diminish over several weeks as you establish new habits of eating less. Initially, though, you just have to put up with some discomfort. Can you binge occasionally as a reward for being "good"? Well, I wouldn't binge, exactly. But you don't have to wear a sackcloth either. You can certainly have cake or ice cream, or some other high-calorie thing, every so often, say once a week, just for fun. But I wouldn't have *a lot* of this stuff at once, nor would I make such an exception more than once a week. As I noted, this is not about torture, but rather about being sensible and reaching a goal.

Managing your fat intake. Of course, some dietary fat is necessary. Fats are part of the steroid-like structure of hormones and a major component of nerve sheaths. Fats are constituents of a transport system that moves proteins and other substances around the body, and they are an important source of energy. Eliminating fat from your diet is unhealthy—we need fat. *Reducing* fat intake is critical to losing weight effectively. About nine or ten years ago I started paying attention to the things I was eating. In the past, I was one of those people who could eat anything and not put on weight. Well, things change. There has been a definite shift in my own metabolic rate as I've gotten older, and I started noticing that my pants were becoming tight around the waist. I was retaining fat! I didn't like this at all; I mean, I used to eat whatever I wanted to eat. For the first time in my life I took a hard look at what I was actually consuming. I was shocked to discover that *fat* represented the bulk of my caloric intake! How could that be? I was thin! But I wasn't as thin as I used to be, and as we discussed previously, you can be an out-of-shape thin person. If I didn't change my dietary habits, that's what I was on the road to becoming.

Exactly what was I eating? Well, I'm a single guy. What do single guys eat? Pizza, peanut butter, ice cream, and takeout. Takeout food, whether Italian or Chinese, is high in saturated fat. My diet was fat, fat, fat. I made broad changes, eliminating pizza and ice cream, switching to reduced-fat peanut butter, and basically managing my calorie intake so that fat represented no more than twenty percent of the total. After about eight weeks I had lost eight pounds or so, and was back to the third notch on my belt. Now eight pounds may not seem like such a big deal, relatively, but it was to me. I didn't like how I felt with that extra weight, and in order to lose it I had to change some long-term eating habits. Since then my weight has remained fairly constant, at about 165 or so. And I've noticed it is easier to put on a few pounds if I'm not regulating my fat consumption. I can put extra butter on that baked potato or eat a pint of ice cream, but I know I'll need to minimize my fat intake for the next week or so. It's a workable balance, and I've worked to get there.

How do you "manage the fat in your diet"? Simply, by reading the nutritional labels on cans and packages. Food nutrients are carbohydrates, proteins, and fat. Carbohydrates and proteins contain 4 calories of energy per gram; fat contains 9 calories per gram. A typical average diet contains about 2000 calories per day. A good fat-maintenance diet is one in which fat represents twenty percent of the calories. So your daily diet should contain no more than 400 calories provided by fat. Since fat contains 9 calories per gram, a good daily dose of fat is less than 45 grams. There are two methods of hitting this target. One is to count your daily fat-gram intake for a week or two, getting a sense of how much fat is contained in the various things you are eating. After about two weeks you don't have to count anymore; you have learned pretty well how much fat is in specific foods. Also, count the total calories. You want to consume 2000 or so calories each day, no more than 400 which are derived from fat. Be sure that you are consuming 45 or less grams of fat per day.

The second method of managing dietary fat is to ensure that fat represents less than 20 percent of the calories contained in each food substance or meal. For example, a 200-calorie energy bar should contain no more than 40 calories provided by fat (about 4.5 grams). If the bar has more than 5 grams of fat, I'll choose another. I want protein and carbohydrates, not fat. In general, food labels state fat quantities in both grams and percentages. The caloric content of a particular item might contain more than 20 percent fat. That's OK, provided that your total daily fat intake is less than 45 grams and the large majority of the things you are eating have caloric contents of less than 20 percent fat. Again, after about two weeks of consistent observation and evaluation of various food products, you'll be able to zoom down the supermarket aisle without having to stop to perform some mental calculations regarding calorie percentages and fat grams. The process becomes automated and easy.

So you do two things. You count the total grams of fat per day and ensure that, for the most part, fat represents no more than 20 percent of the caloric content of each food substance. Here are a number of steps that can assist this process. For canned tuna, use the water-packed rather than oil-packed varieties. Use reduced-fat mayonnaise, peanut butter, and margarine. Buy low-fat ice cream or sorbet, rather than regular ice cream. (I can personally attest that this makes a *huge* difference!) Eat reduced-fat cookies. Eat pretzels (the zero-fat varieties) rather than fatty potato chips. Minimize consumption of dairy products, or choose reduced-fat or low-fat brands. Choose linguini with chicken and broccoli rather than fettucine alfredo (swimming in butter and cream!). And so on. Take the skin off chicken. Minimize things such as bacon and French fries. You get the picture. It takes something to manage this program, but it is really pretty straightforward. There's extra motivation when the pounds start dropping. You'll find you don't want to give up any ground you have already taken, and will want to stick to this new pattern of food consumption.

The last piece in this weight-management puzzle is aerobic exercise. Aerobic exercise is critically important for optimal, healthy functioning. Earlier, when discussing running, we said that aerobic activity causes the heart to become more efficient. The *stroke volume* increases, that is, more blood is pumped during each heartbeat. Since the heart is pumping continuously, increased stroke volume results in significant energy conservation. Also, due to its intrinsic *aerobic* nature, this type of exercise causes fat to be burned for energy. There's less fat in your diet overall, because you're consuming less fat, and simultaneously, you're burning fat because you're doing consistent aerobic exercise. Boom! You're losing weight!

Build up your aerobic activity slowly, as we discussed previously. After about four weeks you should be up to thirty minutes of moderate aerobic exercise, whether it's fast walking, running, stair-climbing, treadmill, or stationary bike. Three times a week is great, four times a week is really great. You may notice that you've lost four or five pounds in these first four weeks. That's a fine start, and keep going! As I said earlier, weight loss is all about intention. Sustainable weight loss results from slow, methodical modification of eating habits and the institution of a consistent, fun, aerobic exercise program. There are no quick solutions. And, everyone can lose the weight they want to lose and maintain their new bodies!

Let's look at the broader topic of nutrition itself. We're going to take the common-sense approach to nutrition. As with exercise, eating effectively requires intentionality. It's a random universe, tending toward entropy (greater disorder), and left alone, most things (humans included) will take the path of least resistance toward a disordered, less-organized state. With regard to nutrition, an "ordered state" would be one in which you are eating a variety of good things from all major food groups. A "disordered" nutritional state, one in which there's less intentionality and less causation, probably would consist of jelly doughnuts, bagels and cream cheese, fast food (hamburgers, Mexican, Chinese, whatever), and frozen pizza. Maybe including the occasional banana. I know for myself that, unless I make a point of it, I could go without vegetables for a *really* long time.

Before extensive urbanization, people ate what was nearby. There was fresh milk and eggs, meat, breads, and fruit and vegetables. There were local slaughterhouses in *Brooklyn!* We had a milkman who delivered milk to our back door! Things change. A lot. Transcontinental and intercontinental delivery of foods into urban centers is commonplace. Some degree of freshness is consistently lost. Animals are given antibiotics and growth hormones to increase production yields. Crops are sprayed with pesticides to minimize losses. OK, this is the world we live in. There's no going back, and we don't want to go back. Not really. In this context, how do we fulfill our nutritional requirements so that our biological machines are maintained, and we're able to do the things we're meant to do as human beings?

The solutions is straightforward. Good nutrition can be obtained without a whole lot of effort. There will be *some* effort, but not too much. Effective nutrition consists in adhering to several *basic* principles. We've noted two of them already: drink a lot of water and manage the fat content of your diet. The third basic principle is to eat consistently and with variety items contained in *all* the major food groups. During the course of a week, consume things that are grain-based; eat a bunch of fruit and vegetables; have some meat, fish, and/or poultry; and possibly consume some milk, yogurt, and/or cheese.

Is that it? Well, there's a lot more to say, but yes, that's pretty much it. We get off track when we don't follow these principles; for the most part, Americans don't follow these principles in the least. The fat content of our diets is way out of line. Over the years, probably nine out of ten of my new patients drink far less than four glasses of water a day. And the food content of our diets is typically skewed toward two of the main groups, causing us to miss out on essential and critical nutrients. So, my suggestion that effective nutrition flows from applying a few basic principles may seem simplistic, but these practices actually work when applied consistently. Simple rules work. As we are learning from the science of complexity, highly complex systems are typically based on a few simple rules. For example, our intricately complex human DNA sequences are composed of only *four* building blocks: adenine, thymine, guanine, and cytosine. Similarly, the complex tissues that comprise a human organism are composed of molecules built out of the food we eat, the air we breathe, and the water we drink. Simple input; complex output. There's no need to complicate the process of eating. Just be sure to eat everything you need, that is, pay attention to consuming things from every food group.

What I'm specifically not discussing here is the *politics* of nutrition: you *should* eat this, or you *shouldn't* eat that. These "natural" things are good for you; these "processed" things are bad for you. I don't subscribe to these "shoulds" and "shouldn'ts". If you have developed a harmonious frame of mind (or at least, *relatively* harmonious!) you will instinctively choose the things that are good for *you.* And, sometimes you won't. I've mentioned my fondness for ice cream. I do go through periods when I am eating a lot of ice cream. Eventually, after I've gained a few pounds, I'll stop and lose that weight again. It's OK. I'm not perfect. But I do have a good knowledge base and know when to stop indulging and return to more healthy eating.

Let's look more closely at instinctively choosing the things that are good for you. How do you get to this state of grace? First, there is the desire to take care of your machine and knowing how to do that. Likewise, you take your car in for regular tune-ups and change the oil in your car's engine periodically. You eat from all four food groups, drink water, and manage the fat in your diet. Pretty much the same kind of thing. Next, you become someone who consistently exercises. Regular exercise creates a need for good nutrition. You need more water, you need more glucose, you need more protein. You need sources of energy to replace the energy expended on activity. New energy comes from eating foods across the spectrum of food groups. If you eat junk your performance will suffer, and if you're paying attention, you will be training yourself to eat effectively. Eating well is a process of course correction, one which ultimately will result in eliminating most of the high-fat, highly processed, high-calorie-low-nutritional-content foods from our diets.

You develop an instinct, one which works for you. I almost never eat pizza now; it used to be one of my major food groups. I don't each quiche, cheesecake (almost never), or cream-based pasta sauces. I never eat from fast-food establishments. I make sure to have fruit and/or vegetables every day. Now, I'm still not that great on vegetables. My vegetables are potatoes, corn, tomatoes, occasionally broccoli, some lettuce-type stuff like romaine and Mesclun. Green vegetables are a weak area for me. Don't offer me Brussels sprouts; don't offer me cauliflower. But I'm not a bad person. My point is my diet is way better than it was when I was completely unintentional about it. My eating is far more well-rounded than in the past. This is my recommendation. *Balanced* eating. Not *fanatical* eating. Good nutrition can be obtained with some modest effort; there's no need to be obsessive and have guilt. Eat ice cream once a week. Have one or two pieces of chocolate, rather than three or five or ten. Reduce fat whenever possible, but yes, you can put sour cream on your baked potato once in a while, as a bonus for being good.

Let's talk about breakfast. I'll repeat here what has been stated many times elsewhere. Breakfast *is* important. Very important. Basically, if you don't eat breakfast you're running on empty. Your brain, the body's biggest consumer of glucose, is temporarily malnourished. You can't possibly be maximally productive in the morning without breakfast. Are you "sluggish" in the morning, "no good until you have your coffee", irritable, cranky? Do you have headaches which begin around 10 or 11 a.m.? What's missing is sufficient glucose for effective brain function. Also, you are metabolizing glycogen to provide needed energy for your body to get from here to there. You are wasting both the energy it took to store excess glucose as glycogen and the energy used to metabolize it because you didn't have breakfast. Simply, skipping breakfast causes your metabolic functions to go through various gyrations to maintain homeostasis. Possible long-term consequences include gastrointestinal irritation, hypoglycemia, and elevated blood pressure, as well as alienated family members, neighbors, and coworkers. So, is it worth it to be intentional, get up fifteen minutes earlier, and eat some fun things for breakfast? If we're interested in maintaining a healthy machine, operating at higher levels of effectiveness, and having more fun, yes, it's worth it.

What might there be for breakfast? Orange juice; whole-grain toast with fruit preserves, low-fat peanut butter, or low-fat cream cheese; an apple or banana; low-fat granola; low-fat or no-fat yogurt; even a hard-boiled egg. Any or all of these. Mix and match. How long does it take to throw such a simple, highly nourishing breakfast together? No time at all. Notice there is neither sausage, bacon, nor home-fried potatoes. We're managing the fat in our diet, beginning with the first meal of the day.

What about milk? Milk is an excellent source of protein; however, milk is not for everybody. Some people are lactose-intolerant; for them, milk is an unpleasant irritant to the lower gastrointestinal tract. Also, milk is probably not an effective food for those individuals who have many allergies or have autoimmune disorders such as rheumatoid arthritis or lupus erythematosus. For everybody else, the primary concern about milk is its fat content. Whole milk contains about nine grams of fat per eight-ounce serving. "Two-percent" milk contains about five grams of fat per eight-ounce serving. Note that "two-percent" milk does not mean that two percent of the calories in an eight-ounce glass are derived from fat. Actually, fat represents almost forty percent of the calories in "two-percent" milk. This doesn't meet our fat-should-be-no-more-than-twenty-percent-of-the-calories-in-a-food rule, but if your total fat intake for the day is still only forty or forty-five grams, a glass of "two-percent" milk fits right in. Skim milk, of course, has zero fat.

What about coffee? Well, I never knew what coffee was about until I started drinking it. I've only been drinking coffee for less than ten years, and when I started I thought, "Oh, this is why people drink coffee". The stimulant effect of caffeine was quite revelatory. My sense here is that, like anything else, coffee done to excess is troublesome. Caffeine causes the kidneys to excrete more water, so there is a dehydrating effect. Of course, caffeine is addictive, creating its own metabolic-endocrine dependency, so this is to be avoided. One cup of coffee per day is completely acceptable and should not generate any guilt or sense of being a nutritional defective. Two cups a day, every day, is probably close to too much. Two cups a day a few times a week is probably reasonable and realistic for most of us. I encourage patients who drink more coffee than this to reduce their intake. I'm not interested in their eliminating coffee as a habit, that will never happen, but rather in modifying their coffee dosage so they regain control. Coffee tastes great and it's fun to drink coffee! In moderation.

What about lunch? Well, the same principles apply. You want to have nutritious things from the major food groups, maintain fat intake at twenty percent or less of the total calories, and avoid "empty" calories (high in sugar and refined carbohydrates). To manage this requires some attention. Ordering from the local delicatessen or coffee shop is the easiest approach, but the nutritional content is likely to be low and the fat content and total calories are likely to be high. One solution is to find a local nutrition-oriented takeout place that has a variety of fresh entrées, sandwiches, and salads. These establishments usually have a terrific selection of juice drinks and shakes. For example, you can have a whole-grain sandwich with chicken or turkey, providing complex carbohydrates and protein, and a shake providing more carbohydrates in the form of fruit and/or vegetables. Nutrition goal accomplished! If you search a little you can find a nearby restaurant that provides a breakdown of the calorie content, fat grams, and protein grams for their pastas and other nutritious entrées.

A second solution is to bring lunch to work. This is not as bad as it might sound, and you could bring lunch some days and order takeout or eat out other days. A typical lunch I bring to my office includes tuna-and-tomato on whole-grain bread (six-ounce can of tuna packed in water, mixed with a teaspoon of low-fat mayonnaise—6 grams of fat for the sandwich), a banana, and three pretzels (zero fat, 100 calories and 3 grams of protein per pretzel). If I add a cup of non-fat yogurt, that's another 110 calories and 7 grams of protein. That's a heck of a lunch! Of course, I'm drinking plenty of water during the day at work. So, it's easy to bring lunch to work. It just takes a little preparation in terms of shopping and putting the items together. The benefits include total control, complete knowledge of the ingredients and nutritional content, and the convenience of having your lunch already with you, which may save 15 to 30 minutes of valuable time.

These composition and content guidelines are also applicable to dinner. One concern is the time of the evening meal. In days gone by, families usually had dinner at 6 p.m. or so. Most people I know have their last meal of the day at 7:30, 8:30, or even 9 p.m. The concern is that this is too late, you go to bed soon thereafter, and rather than burning up the calorie content, the calories are converted to fat because the body is resting. This would be so, except for two main points. First, you're managing the fat content of your diet, and second, you're exercising consistently. Here's a key point about exercise: exercise builds lean muscle mass and simultaneously increases your body's basal metabolic rate. You burn more calories, even while you are resting, to satisfy the metabolic demands of the streamlined muscle tissue. So, whereas an 8:30 dinner time may not be ideal in terms of calorie utilization, it will work for you provided your weekly schedule contains three good exercise sessions. Exercise and diet should enrich your life, rather than forcing you to attempt unworkable lifestyle alterations to meet inflexible "healthy" commandments. The latter scenario will not happen in reality. So, some shifts in habits will probably be necessary to accommodate a new nutritional focus, but these will be choices *you* have made and they will be choices that are empowering.

What about vitamins and other nutritional supplements? It's easy and appropriate to conclude that daily vitamin/mineral supplementation is useful and probably necessary. Of course, I've been taking daily "vitamins" since the age of six, so for me it's the habit of a lifetime. I'm used to it and doing so always made sense to me, even during my tumultuous 1960s adolescence. The purpose of supplementation is to cover all bases, to make sure they are covered. It would take a *lot* of work to be certain that your diet contained sufficient iodine, magnesium, selenium, chromium, folate, and vitamins B_1 (thiamin), B_2 (riboflavin), B_3 (niacin), B_6 (pyridoxine), and B_{12} (cyanocobalamin). Taking a supplement guarantees that daily vitamin and mineral requirements have been met. It's simple, safe, and efficient in terms of both time and cost.

Which brand of supplementation is best? There's no right answer here, it's more of an instinctive decision. About five years ago I changed brands, switching from a mass-market product I had been purchasing in a health-food store to a specialty, designer-type product available by mail order. My experience was that, overall, I was more rested and had more energy than previously. In a word, I was "peppier", and the only variable that had altered was switching to a new brand of supplements. Recently, I switched back to a mass-market brand and found my subjective results just as good. The claims of both products are similar: the minerals are chelated, which presumably facilitates their absorption from the digestive tract as opposed to their being excreted as waste. The refining processes use filtered water; the source materials are "natural" foods.

My sense is that there is no real, clinically demonstrable difference between these designer products. In fact, there may be no real quantitative difference between these brands and the mass-market labels on the shelves of your local store. Choose a brand, take it for four weeks, and if you like how you "feel", stay with that product. Brand selection is instinctive. Brand selection is personal. There are no peer-reviewed, hard statistical data suggesting that one brand is superior. "Results" here are qualitative, not quantitative. The important point is that vitamin/mineral supplementation is necessary to ensure optimal metabolic functioning and physical well-being.

What about using specific supplements for specific things, such as taking calcium supplements after a bone-density study has revealed loss of bone mass (osteoporosis)? Is this an effective therapy? The observable fact is that a loss of bone mass has occurred. Bone mass consists of bone cells and bone matrix. Bone cells are called osteoblasts. Bone matrix contains protein and hydroxyapatite, a compound composed of calcium and phosphate. So, yes, there has been a loss of calcium in osteoporosis. But let's look at this in more detail. Attempting to replace this depleted calcium by taking oral supplements is an action based on the most superficial interpretation of the pathophysiology. There are a number of analytical and logical errors that lead to such an approach. Osteoporosis frequently occurs in menopausal women, in part due to a loss of estrogen production. Estrogen stimulates osteoblast activity; decreased osteoblast activity results in decreased bone production. Taking oral calcium at this point will not increase bone mass. The point of failure is not lack of calcium, per se, but rather a decrease in the overall production of bone.

Bone mass will only be added if there is a physiologic demand for such an increase, that is, if there is sufficient *stress* on bone to necessitate strengthening the existing bony structures. Such an increase in stress occurs with exercise. Wolff's law (a physiologic principle) states that bone remodels along lines of physiologic stress. Exercise causes long bones to bear increased mechanical loads during relatively short intervals: the normal physiologic response is to stimulate osteoblast activity to build new bone. Conversely, if you are not exercising, not challenging the physical structure of your bones, the normal physiologic response is to remove calcium and other valuable minerals from bone that could be better used elsewhere. The human body conserves its resources in remarkable ways. Simply, use it or lose it.

Several points can now be made. Consistent exercise, in the context of really paying attention to physical health, is relatively new in our society. It is likely that the great majority of older people (let's define this group as over age 60) did not do much exercise for most of their adult lives. Since bone densitometry is a relatively new procedure, implying that earlier comparison studies are not available for many women, it's possible that the finding of loss of bone mass relates as much to lack of exercise as to lack of estrogen.

Another point relates to the purpose and value of calcium supplementation. In the postmenopausal setting, if you're not exercising, the calcium taken orally will simply be excreted. Completely useless. On the other hand, if you are exercising or begin an exercise program, the additional calcium may be useful in providing raw material for osteoblast activity—raw material for new bone formation, created in response to the stress of exercise. What about calcium supplementation for younger women? Again, exercise is the key to forestalling osteoporosis. Of course, this is in the context of sufficient calcium intake. The recommended daily requirement for calcium is 1000 mg. My vitamin/mineral supplement supplies 500 mg. If I have a cup of yogurt, that's another 250 mg. A glass of skim milk (zero fat) or a piece of low-fat cheese adds another 250 mg, and I'm set for the day! Non-dairy sources of calcium include calcium-fortified orange juice, spinach, turnips, and sardines (with the bones). So, dietary sources plus your vitamin/mineral supplements provide sufficient daily calcium. Additional calcium tablets or pills are often not necessary. Since the body does not store calcium, as such, if you're taking oral calcium, the excess is excreted.

Laboratory diagnosis, one of the topics I teach in the orthopedics board-certification program for chiropractors, is a notoriously difficult subject. The facts are not intuitive; there are no simple explanations. "Why" is a question that is asked repetitively and sequentially as deeper and deeper layers of answers are given. Laboratory diagnosis evaluates biochemical and metabolic processes, complex events whose interactions are intricately interwoven. Event A is caused by event B, which may be caused by event C or event D, which in turn is caused by events E, F, or G, and so on. There are almost no simple, direct relationships in biochemistry/metabolism or, said another way, physiology. Event X is rarely caused only by event Y.

Nutrition is a practical application of the studies of physiology, biochemistry, and metabolism. Consider this. Element Z is reduced or missing in a certain individual who manifests condition Q. Since biochemical/metabolic interactions are linked by a cascading series of events, it would be naïve to think that supplying element Z would solve condition Q. Yet, this is exactly what is proposed in recommendations to purchase this or that nutritional element, whether calcium, tryptophan, zinc, or folic acid. Can these substances be useful? Yes. Can they provide benefit? Yes, frequently.

However, what about all the other elements that are part of the cascade of events leading to condition Q? How deep an analysis has been conducted? Is it possible that supplying excess quantities of element Z will distort other variables in the cascade, causing unforeseen, new problems? What if element Z is almost irrelevant to the problem, that is, Z is reduced because of a malfunction in system S? And so on. Thus, the usefulness and effectiveness of recommending individual supplemental substances are similar to the accuracy with which the three blind men describe the elephant: the one holding the tail says the elephant is narrow and thin like a hairy rope; the one with his arms wrapped around the elephant's leg says the animal is shaped like a tree and covered with leathery bark; and the one holding the trunk says the elephant reminds him of a snake with a puckering mouth. The complete elephant, with all its complex and contrasting components, has not been perceived.

Of course, in the treatment of specific medical conditions, specific missing ingredients can be key: vitamin D in the case of rickets, vitamin B_1 for beri-beri, vitamin B_3 for pellagra, vitamin B_{12} for macrocytic anemia, vitamin K for hemophilia, and so on. However, for the vast majority of the population, specific nutrient supplementation may be necessary only in the short term, to return to a baseline level of health. For most of

us, a well-rounded diet and a daily vitamin/mineral supplement are sufficient to maintain good health over the long term.

This brings us back to being personally responsible for how our lives
are going. If I'm not sleeping well, is it because I'm missing the amino acid
tryptophan in my diet, or are there issues and concerns in my life that I
am not addressing authentically and directly? Probably the latter is more
accurate. If I'm sluggish and fatigued, do I need to take ginseng capsules
or tea, or some other "natural" product to pep me up? Or could I take a
look at what's not working in my life, possibly acknowledging that I
haven't exercised, gone to a museum, or called my mother in years. I suggest that physical breakdowns and personal breakdowns are closely
related. I don't mean this to be the *truth*. I propose this hypothesis as a
springboard to initiating an inquiry into the circumstances of one's life.
The key question of such an inquiry is *what is missing?*

It's typical for us to look outside ourselves for answers to physical
problems and health concerns. Fatigue, malaise, depleted energy, lack of
restful sleep, and gastrointestinal disorders are common problems that
cause people to seek "nutritional" solutions. I'll assert that most of these
disorders will not be solved "out there" by taking various specific
substances. More effective healing is obtained by an inner search,
conducted as an inquiry: Who am I? What is my life for? What's happening
in my relationships with family, friends, and colleagues? What messes have
I made and what is there to clean up? What have I been avoiding? What is
missing? What empowers me, and what, in contrast, have I been
empowering instead? Who do I choose to be?

The answers that flow from these internal investigations will create a
context for a healthy, happy, fully realized life. But there may be pressing
concerns. How can we address the actual physical dysfunctions that are
present *today?* The primary solution is for me to take control of my life: I
am responsible. My circumstances are my circumstances, and I am still
responsible for how my life goes. I can take responsibility in the arena of
health by initiating or returning to a consistent exercise program, being

sure I eat a well-rounded diet, managing the fat in my diet, and taking daily vitamin/mineral supplements. Over time, to the extent that I am willing to *be* a healthy person, these physical dysfunctions will resolve. My sleep is rested, I have plenty of energy, my skin is clear, and my gastrointestinal system does what it is designed to do.

An additional valuable practice in the ongoing creation of vibrant health is that of daily meditation. In the past, when someone recommended meditation to me, I would imagine myself sitting cross-legged on the floor, with a straight back, repetitively chanting the word "Om". This was an unpleasant image—I associated meditation with discomfort, knee pain, and back pain. Also, I wondered how I could sit perfectly still for any length of time. How could I concentrate for the duration required? I never saw any way I could *do* meditation successfully. I made some half-hearted attempts here and there and always quit, experiencing the process as difficult, uncomfortable, and boring.

Years ago my brother began practicing Transcendental Meditation, and he told me about a number of remarkable health benefits he experienced. Of course, he recommended the method, but I was still stuck in my interpretation of what meditation "was" and did not act on his advice. Three years ago I was reading a wonderful book on health and healing in which the author described TM in detail. He made many points about the health benefits flowing from the practice of TM, citing twenty-five years of peer-reviewed research which quantified those results. He specifically noted that older people who begin TM test "younger" in relation to various physiologic parameters, when compared to matched controls who are not meditating. This retardation-of-aging effect is magnified as the practice continues over time. Well, finally, that was all I needed to know! I thought, *I'm getting older!* Apparently, here's a powerful tool specifically designed to support human physiology. There's hard, peer-reviewed data to prove it. *Get going!* Well, self-interest became more powerful than prejudice. Instruction in transcendental meditation takes only a few short lessons. I learned how to meditate and have been practicing TM for more than three years. It is simple, straightforward, practical, highly effective, and rewarding.

TM is truly easy. You meditate for twenty minutes, twice a day. Twenty minutes in the morning, and twenty minutes in the late afternoon or early evening. There's no breathing pattern, and there's no chanting. There are no awkward positional requirements. You sit comfortably in a chair or on a sofa. You close your eyes and begin silently repeating a mantra, a couple of meaningless syllables you're given during your instruction. That's it. You keep repeating the mantra. Of course, the mantra is not exactly continuous. Other thoughts intrude, and you gently remind yourself to go back to repeating the syllables of the mantra. These syllables have no meaning, per se, but the sounds are designed to have specific physiologic effects. Apparently, beginning the mantra is like pushing a button on an automatic mechanism. Once you're engaged in the process of repeating the mantra, whatever happens, happens. For example, you didn't have a "bad" session if you were thinking a lot of thoughts. If for some unusual reason you need to interrupt your meditation, you pick it up later and complete those twenty minutes.

It's an easy, relaxed experience. If you have to scratch your nose, do so. The only "requirement" is to do two twenty-minute sessions per day. There is no benefit obtained if you do less than this. What's going on in TM? Well, the process provides deep rest, both physical and mental. I noted several immediate and unexpected responses to my initial practice of TM. First, surprisingly, I observed that my workouts were easier, requiring less *effort*. Now, I've been training for more than thirty years, it's not like it's anything new. Sometimes it's hard work. But I found that much of the *work* had been removed and there was much less fatigue, or no fatigue, afterward. I was impressed. Similarly, I experienced more of a *flow* in my creative activities. The process of writing became smoother; I had gained quicker access to *ideas*. Reading was facilitated as well; I noticed an increase in my reading rate. Also, I found that I was paying more acute attention to music and to visual stimuli.

Physically, I've had a good several years. TM has been an important part of this result. I can't quantify the benefits, I was healthy when I started, but the experiential effects are of great value *and* health-wise I'm very well. The profound physiologic rest provided by TM is energizing. It's like recharging your battery. What could you accomplish if your fuel cells were fully charged, ongoingly? This is the opportunity of TM.

There are a few other things to discuss in the arena of nutrition. You've noticed I've said nothing so far about vegetarianism or fasting. My sense is that if one or both methods work for you, that's fine. I have no agenda here. I don't say it's necessary to eat meat, but I'm certainly not going to suggest that there's anything wrong with doing so. Similarly, I'm not a vegetarian, but I'm not going to suggest that a person needs meat products to ensure a well-rounded diet. What is of concern is maintaining a complete diet in terms of essential nutrients. People who eat vegetarian diets need to pay special attention to obtaining requisite amounts of protein.

On average, protein should constitute about fifteen percent of your daily caloric intake. If you're consuming 2000 calories per day, that's 300 calories provided by protein. At four calories per gram of protein, that's 75 grams of protein per day. What food sources might supply this amount of protein? For a vegetarian diet, four slices of whole-grain bread provide 16 grams of protein, a cup of beans (kidney, lima, or lentil) provides 15 grams, one cup of rice provides 15 grams, four ounces of tofu provide 10 grams, two tablespoons of peanut butter provide 8 grams, three zero-fat pretzels provide 9 grams, and a cup of soy milk provides 9 grams, for a total of 82 grams. A good day's worth of protein!

It's important to consume foods containing *essential* amino acids, those protein constituents that humans do not produce physiologically. Protein sources supplying all the essential amino acids are considered *complete*. Milk, dairy products, fish, and meat supply complete protein. In vegetarian diets, tofu, soy milk, and tempeh contain all the essential amino acids. Also, combining rice and beans or other grains and beans provides *complete* protein.

Thus, a vegetarian diet is a healthy one provided it contains sufficient and complete protein. What I am specifically not saying is that such a diet is intrinsically "healthier" than a meat-containing diet. There is no proof of this assertion, one way or another. As with every other health-related issue, my approach is empiric. What works, works. You evaluate what is "working", in the absence of quantifiable, reproducible data, by assessing your experience. Do I feel better or worse, doing this or that? Am I more energized, invigorated, focused, productive when I eat a balanced diet containing meat products? Or are these states occurring when I concentrate my diet toward the vegetarian end of things? It's a personal call, and your habits and choices may change over the years, back and forth. The challenge to clear thinking in this area derives from sociocultural overlays of what is considered "enlightened" behavior, none of which has anything to do with scientific inquiry.

The late composer, Toru Takemitsu, said, "When sounds are possessed by ideas instead of having their own identity, music suffers". Likewise with health-related concerns. Any social bias distorts objective discourse. There is no intrinsic "rightness" about including or excluding meat and/or dairy products from your diet. Really, whatever works for you is the way to go, as distinct from what someone says you "should" do. If you wish to avoid the antibiotics, hormones, and other stimulants/suppressants given to cattle, swine, and poultry, that's fine, and it might even be appropriate to do so. But I'm not necessarily making an "unhealthy" choice if I continue to buy such food from my regular butcher. Might it be better to seek out more "natural" meat and poultry products, derived from animals grown in a less "supplemented" environment? Probably. But there's no need to be obsessive about this search. There's simply no uncontested data supporting any of these points of view. Make dietary choices that are empowering, ones that support your concepts of health and well-being. And please remember that your choices may not necessarily be those of another, who is making the choices that empower him or her.

What about "juice fasts" and other forms of fasting? Do these regimens provide necessary "detoxification"? I really don't know. There are no proofs in this area; only non-reproducible data are available, mostly in the form of case reports and subjective experiences. I offer no recommendations here, but if you choose to fast, do so with supervision. Importantly, are there any factors in your medical history, such as heart disease or diabetes, that would be exacerbated by such a program? What are your intended outcomes of the fast? Why are you doing it? Make an informed decision.

Earlier, I mentioned the "ongoing creation of vibrant health". As with any other system in our corner of the universe, disorder will prevail over order whenever order is not maintained intentionally. Dust balls accumulate, desk drawers are filled with junk, piles of paper spread from the desk to the dining room table to the floor, your car's underbody rusts, and your new computer's hard disk access time gets longer and longer. Machines maintain their functionality and performance over time when they receive regular maintenance. Junk (randomness) proliferates in the environment unless periodic cleaning, filing, arranging, and disposal occurs. Likewise with human health.

Junk (arteriosclerotic plaquing) builds up unless specific steps are taken in the areas of aerobic exercise and fat maintenance. Disorder (in the form of replacement of highly specialized muscle fibers with low-grade, non-contractile connective tissue) prevails in the absence of exercise. What do we choose to do about all this? Well, being healthy is a choice. If I choose to be healthy, OK, terrific, and here are the things to do to support that choice: exercise, fat management, good nutrition, being present in the world. Each of these requires intentionality. There will be times when I am not intentional, and disorder sets in as a consequence. I'm human, not perfect, and I will stumble along the way. All there is to do is to get back in action. The key is to get back in action *with velocity.* Give up ice cream, again. Go back to the gym, again. Why? Because I choose to, because I choose health.

And if I don't, that's OK too, but I should not be surprised by the effects of my choices. Now, most of us know someone who has smoked cigarettes all his life and is still chugging along, pretty vibrantly, in his eighties. Or the person who has "never exercised" who is seventy-five and enviably slim. We may also know someone who was a runner for many years and who suffered a massive heart attack at the age of forty-five. Stuff happens. There are always exceptions. Still, it would be unusual to expect a sports car to continue functioning well without regular service. The bottom line is who are you, what do you intend to accomplish, and what will support you in being that and getting there? I suggest that vibrant, dynamic physical health will support a person in all his or her endeavors. And, the creation of health is an ongoing process, one that is never complete. It really is a journey.

With respect to the nutritional component of dynamic health, I'll reiterate that the best nutritional program is based on common sense, and common sense can be applied when a good fund of basic knowledge is available. The rules of nutrition are simple: ensure a balanced diet; consume appropriate amounts of carbohydrate, protein, and fat; in general, manage the fat in your diet; take a daily vitamin/mineral supplement; and drink a lot of water. There is some work involved in this, some attention to details. The benefits are considerable.

CHAPTER 9

▼

"TRUST ME, I'M A DOCTOR": CREATING A DOCTOR/PATIENT PARTNERSHIP

What do we do when something goes wrong with our physical machine? Of course, there's a range of choices, but often the easiest action is *inaction*. The human body has remarkable recuperative powers, and time and rest will solve many problems. Many other situations require professional attention: you have acute, intense pain; you have nagging pain that won't go away or is getting worse; or you may have long-term, lingering pain or discomfort that has become an annoyance and you want it fixed. [Our discussion here will focus on disturbances of the musculoskeletal system (bones, joints, ligaments, muscles, and tendons) and is not intended to address diseases of other systems, such as the respiratory, gastrointestinal, or endocrine systems.] What are our professional choices? In other words, which type of practitioner should be consulted for which types of problems? Specialists in the world of fitness, in the context of having a body that works, include chiropractors, orthopedic surgeons, physical therapists, physiatrists (doctors of physical medicine), osteopaths, and bodyworkers in various disciplines.

Each specialty offers a specific form of treatment; also, there are broad areas of overlap between, for example, chiropractors, physiatrists, and physical therapists. Some conditions are best handled by a particular discipline. Also, each specialty has its strengths and limitations; there is no "best" type of doctor or therapist. However, there are "best" methods of examination, diagnosis, and treatment: these "best practices" are found in all the physical medicine disciplines. I'd like to discuss chiropractic at length, since my experience and expertise are in that field. Later, we'll evaluate optimal strategies for restoring health and function, utilizing the best available methods from all therapeutic systems.

Chiropractic physicians are specialists in the diagnosis and treatment of musculoskeletal disorders, specifically those involving biomechanical dysfunction: muscle strains, ligament sprains, restricted mobility, radiating arm and leg pain, numbness and tingling of the extremities, disc injuries, and many types of headaches. Like any other physician, a chiropractor takes a full history and performs a physical examination in his specialty, including orthopedic, neurologic, and biomechanical evaluation. Other studies may be ordered, including x-rays and blood tests. A differential diagnosis is developed, rank-ordering the several most likely causes of the particular person's problem. Having determined that the person is in the right place, that is, has a problem that can be successfully addressed by chiropractic treatment and that there are no contraindications to such an approach, a treatment plan is designed. The most typical method of addressing biomechanical disorders is joint manipulative therapy, most often spinal manipulative therapy.

Before we examine what joint manipulation is, I'd like to look at a few things that may be in the background when we talk about chiropractic. A new patient might express to me his concern that "once you start seeing a chiropractor you have to go for the rest of your life". Or "I don't want to get hooked on chiropractic". Well, I don't want you to get hooked, either. In fact, most chiropractic cases can be handled in the short term. The goals of treatment are to reduce and/or resolve pain, return to function, restore previous levels of fitness by reestablishing an exercise program, and learn techniques and procedures (lifestyle modification, physical activities) that keep a person healthy. Some cases can be resolved in one to three visits, others may require up to ten visits or so. The large majority of new patients should be managed on this basis. The minority of cases, those that are either more acutely severe or more lingering and chronic, require more extended treatment plans. The goal should always be to end acute treatment and discharge the person, having trained the individual in both the stretching procedures and rehabilitative exercises that will keep them well.

Be proactive when choosing a chiropractic physician, as you would when selecting a surgeon, electrician, or investment advisor. Ask questions. How long does it take to get the average new patient well? Ten to twelve visits is a good median, representing both the one-to-three-visit cases and the more chronic, twenty- to thirty-visit cases. Is the chiropractor expert in the treatment and prevention of sports-related injuries? Has he or she taken postgraduate education in this area? Does he or she consistently utilize rehabilitative exercise in the management of patients? Does the chiropractor develop a *differential diagnosis* for each case? These few questions will provide a quick, useful profile of that particular physician's expertise.

At the conclusion of the initial evaluation (history taking and physical examination), your chiropractor should briefly outline the following: *working diagnosis*, possible additional testing, methods of treatment, and anticipated outcomes. The working diagnosis is the most likely diagnosis based on the available information; it represents the most probable of a list of diagnostic entities that might fit the specific information. This list comprises the *differential diagnosis*. The differential diagnosis is a rank-ordered list of several potential causes of a person's condition, ranging from probable to possible. A well-conceived list includes four to six specific entities or categories of conditions; such a list will almost always represent 98+% of the possible causes of a person's ailment. Rarer, unlikely causes are simply that: they are rare and will be considered if treatment for the more typical conditions has not been successful. Of course, if a rare condition is suggested by the data it will be included on the differential list and addressed in the early stages of evaluation.

When I speak with a new patient I'll say something like, "The working diagnosis here is 'X'." I might mention a statistical likelihood related to this conclusion. ("Based on the available data I have 95% confidence in this diagnosis.") I may add, "We're still going to consider "Y", and if we haven't made some improvement within five days or so, we'll proceed with further evaluation. Does this recommendation make sense? Do you have any questions about what I've just said?" This allows the person to partic-ipate in the management of their care and provides an opportunity for fur-ther discussion.

Here are the most typical causes of lower back pain, as an example of a differential diagnosis. The first two are the most common: biomechanical or musculoskeletal dysfunction or injury (including strains, sprains, and limited joint mobility), herniated disc material irritating a spinal nerve, spinal stenosis (narrowing of the canal that contains the spinal cord), radiating pain from organic disease (for example, kidney or pancreatic inflammation), and tumor (benign or malignant). The minority of the causes of lower back pain, including organic disease and tumor, are scary and serious, but are present, overall, in less than five percent of cases.

Serious causes of pain should *always* be *considered* in evaluating a case; for the most part they are ruled out (eliminated as a possibility) by the physical examination. So—you choose a chiropractor or other specialist based not only on his ability to treat, but possibly more importantly, on his ability to make an accurate diagnosis. Whenever improvement is not being obtained after a reasonable period of time, the case needs to be reevaluated and other, less typical, causes of the problem investigated.

How can a businesswoman, an artist, a teamster, or a policeman evaluate a physician's skills? By asking questions. Not asking questions for their own sake, but to get a sense of the individual in whom you are entrusting your health. Often it is not necessary to ask: the doctor's manner, approach, and ability to communicate address the patient's unasked questions. In other situations, being direct is best: "Doctor, I have a concern." Or, "Doctor, will we be addressing this possibility?" Or, "How can I help myself get better quickly?" The replies to your questions will help you choose whether this particular office is the place to be.

I support the concept of full disclosure from the doctor to the patient. This is not to say that each person needs to know every little fact and detail. For example, I never discuss particular named diseases with people, unless I believe the question *needs* to be addressed or I am specifically asked. If I request that a person go for laboratory tests or I recommend consultation with a neurologist or internist, a person might ask, "Doc, what do you think it is?" Or, "What are you looking for?" There are no good answers to a question like this. Of course, we are looking to rule out something serious, some disease or condition that is still in the running after the history and physical exam have been done. Most people realize that x-rays are matter-of-fact, standard procedures, but lab tests or referrals cause alarms to go off.

Another question is, "Is this serious?" Most people are well informed. They're not physicians, not specialists, but much basic medical information is now generally available. Football analysts talk about knee reconstructions—repair of the "ACL, MCL, and patellar tendon"—in casual analysis of the factors contributing to a particular game outcome. Movie and television stars discuss their diseases and surgeries on talk shows. Prime-time medical dramas lead the TV ratings. People know what's going on. And, yes, it's important to share the information I have.

But, in my experience it's not helpful to say "what I'm looking for". The person worries, gets scared, and may be angry when the tests come back negative. Thus, my response to such inquiries is, "You know, I appreciate your concern. And there's no good answer to your question right now. I've learned never to outline the possibilities until I have all the information. When the test results are in we'll go over everything together. Is that OK?" I can't do anything to allay a person's fears. I certainly don't want to amplify or exacerbate his concerns. I'm clear in my communication, the person is satisfied that the bases are being covered, and we'll review the case and make recommendations on the follow-up visit.

Once it has been established that yes, you are a candidate for chiropractic treatment, your chiropractor should describe the specific methods of treatment and the anticipated outcomes. There are three main treatment methods utilized by chiropractic physicians: joint manipulative therapy, physical therapeutic modalities, and rehabilitative exercise. Any or all may be utilized in a specific case. I'd like to talk about joint manipulation in some detail.

A person might say, "I went to my chiropractor and she cracked my neck". Or, "My chiropractor cracks my back". I don't know about you, but I'd be pretty apprehensive about going to a doctor who "cracked" any part of my anatomy. What exactly are these people talking about? "Popping" or "cracking" may be heard and/or felt by a person during the joint manipulation. The sounds and sensations are meaningless, they're not the goal of the treatment, but in the absence of any information to the contrary, the patient may experience them as *tangible* results. What are the popping (or "cracking") sounds? Here's a brief description.

When joint ranges of motion are reduced (creating a host of biomechanical disturbances, generally initiating the sequence of events that brought you to the chiropractor's office), blood gases accumulate in the joint space. Normally these gases diffuse back and forth across the capillary–joint interface, propelled back into the circulation by joint motion. With more limited motion there's a relative accumulation of gas molecules within the joint cavity. The forces utilized in manipulation (even though quite small) *cavitate* the gases in the joint, creating presssure on the gases and causing the molecules to rapidly flow across the gap, back into the circulation. The physical result is a popping sound.

Now, what is joint manipulation, why is it utilized, and what are the benefits of this type of treatment? Joint manipulation is a gentle, painless procedure designed to improve joint ranges of motion. What does not occur during chiropractic treatment is putting a bone that was "out of place" "back in place". Nor are spinal bones being "realigned". Physiologically, bones cannot be moved from here to there. No one has a spine that is "out of alignment". During manipulation a joint is brought to the limit of its current range of motion (which is, by definition, less movement than is optimal). The manipulative thrust moves the joint into the *paraphysiologic space,* and now greater movement, closer toward normal, is available. This procedure may be accompanied by a popping sound.

What does the increased joint mobility provide? Here's a short course in biomechanics. Muscle–tendon units move bones; ligaments hold bones together to form joints. Decreased mobility creates mechanical strain on the local soft tissues (muscles and ligaments). Mechanical loads may be taken up at other locations, adding stress to those subsystems. Physically we have wide tolerance limits and remarkable adaptive qualities, but left uncorrected the mechanical system will eventually fail and the person will experience pain. A person might be fine, bend over to pick up a toothbrush or put on socks, and experience excruciating lower back pain. The system failed acutely, very likely representing the endpoint of that person's ability to adapt to deficient biomechanics. Joint manipulation improves joint mobility, bringing it closer toward normal. More normal motion reduces irritative mechanical stresses on muscle–tendon units and ligaments. Loads are balanced and weights are distributed efficiently and effectively. One tangible result is soft-tissue healing and decreased frequency and intensity of pain.

I'd like to discuss a little neurophysiology here. Joint *mechanoreceptors* inform the brain of the exact position of a joint in three dimensions. Mechanoreceptors are also present in muscles, relaying information to the brain about muscle distensibility, tension, and load. How do you know how much force to exert when picking up your twenty-five-pound, eighteen-month-old daughter? Or how much pressure to place on the gas pedal to increase your speed to sixty-five miles per hour? Or how fast to run to reach the drop shot that your tennis opponent has just dumped over the net?

All these calculations are done based on information received from mechanoreceptors. Mechanoreceptor function is impeded in the presence of reduced joint mobility. There is an ensuing loss of information directed centrally, toward the brain, with a resultant loss of optimum physical performance. Bending over to tie your shoelaces is no longer a simple, coordinated act. Feedback of accurate information is disrupted and muscle spasm and pain may result. Or the simple act of twisting your torso to wave goodbye to a friend may result in a similar spasm and pain. In the absence of precise, instantaneous data the biomechanical system will break down.

Mechanoreceptors assist in another important process, that of modulating the conscious experience of pain. Mechanoreceptors assist in a *gating control mechanism:* the gating mechanism dampens pain signals as they're being transmitted to lower centers of the brain. Pain signals may originate from an interaction with external stimuli, for example, touching a hot iron or stubbing your toe on a tree stump. Pain may also originate in internal organs, frequently as a result of a disease process. External pain signals are carried by specialized nerve cells known as *nociceptors.* Much of the "pain" information that stimulates nociceptors is irrelevant; if you were aware of all the "painful" stimuli impacting your body surface you would cease to function effectively. You could not sit in a chair, nor wear clothes. You would be aware of every pressure and touch. There would be signal overload. Mechanoreceptor signals limit the flow of nociceptor signals via the gating control apparatus. Normal mechanoreceptor (joint receptor) function drastically limits the flow of pain signals that reach consciousness.

So, if joint mobility is compromised, the gating mechanism which dampens pain signals is similarly disabled, and you begin to experience pain of which you were not previously aware and which you should not normally experience. This pain can cause a muscular reflex response known as *splinting:* splinting is a muscle spasm designed to limit mobility, reducing further insult to a painful area. A positive feedback loop is established, reinforcing itself with each cycle: reduced joint mobility, altered mechanoreceptor function, enabled pain response, pain, muscle spasm, further reduced joint mobility, and so on.

Joint manipulation intervenes in this cycle by restoring mobility. Mechanoreceptor function is normalized, the gating control mechanism is restored, pain and muscle spasm are reduced and, over time, maximum resolution is obtained. Manipulation is a powerful method for treatment of biomechanical and musculoskeletal problems.

Although critically important, manipulation is not sufficient to fully restore a person's health and well-being. Other key elements, of course, are rest, diet, exercise, and mental attitude. Exercise is a critical part of chiropractic treatment. If you are only receiving manipulative therapy and not exercising, you will improve up to the limit of your current conditioning and no further. On the other hand, if you experience various biomechanical breakdowns and are only exercising, you will improve up to the limit of your biomechanical restraints. Breakdowns will continue to occur until more normal joint mobility is restored by manipulation. The combination of joint manipulative therapy and specific exercise provides for a relatively rapid return to full function. All of my patients receive exercise recommendations, in the context of what is needed for recovery and what that person will actually get up and do.

By the way, joint manipulation describes a variety of procedures. Manipulation can refer to range-of-motion techniques, known as *mobilization,* and also to rapid, rotational movements utilized in the neck and lower back to bring a joint to the limit of its motion and then slightly beyond that limit, as described above. All of these methods are gentle and painless. The mobilization procedures are quite gentle and soothing, almost rhythmic in quality. Again, the purpose is to maximize joint range of motion; mobilization does this by moving the region (neck or lower back) through its various functional planes. Over the last several years I have utilized various mobilization procedures on an increasing basis. I've developed a number of new mobilization methods and use them preferentially for many patients when manipulation would not be appropriate. Of course, the skilled physician has many strings to his bow and will use whatever method is necessary to improve the status of his patient. Medicine is empiric.

I've been treating a woman named Jane for about a year. Jane is one of my longer-term cases. She's in her early fifties and is a short person. Jane is about 4'9" or so and has a very short neck. In fact, she has Klippel-Feil syndrome, a condition in which the vertebras of the neck are maldeveloped. There aren't enough neck bones, some of them are joined together, and others have not achieved their full height. The main consequence of this condition is neck pain and stiffness, which Jane has had her whole adult life. In order to look to the right or left she needs to turn her whole torso in that direction. Essentially, Jane had suffered for years before she began chiropractic treatment. Mobilization was the procedure of choice here, a gentle technique that would restore mobility to a rigid structure in a gradual, stepwise fashion. Over time, hard, knotty bands of muscle in Jane's neck have relaxed and lengthened. Mobility has improved by more that fifty percent. Jane can actually turn her head without turning her torso. The quality of her life has improved substantially; a constant, debilitating irritation has been reduced.

Hilda is an eighty-two-year-old woman whom I treat occasionally for neck spasms. The adjective *dynamic* is not sufficient to describe Hilda. She and her husband have a full social life, in addition to her activities in the artistic and literary communities. Hilda experiences what is termed *torticollis,* a severe neck spasm in which the head is twisted and rotated to one side, almost immobile in that position. Again, mobilization procedures are the optimal treatment choices. After two or three treatments that gradually reduce the muscle spasm and increase joint motion, Hilda returns to normal.

In some cases, I'll begin with mobilization and proceed to manipulation. With obstetric cases I'll use a combination of techniques. Women who are pregnant may develop lower back pain and/or radiating pain into one leg. Here, mobilization involves a gentle, rocking motion over the lower back and pelvis, lengthening the lower back musculature and restoring mobility to the lumbar vertebras and particularly the sacroiliac joints. I'll follow this with manipulation to dynamically increase biomechanical function.

Having described several possible treatment methods, your chiropractor will then discuss expected outcomes of therapy, that is, what results can be anticipated and in what time frames. Each case is unique, of course, but general guidelines are usually applicable. If I'm speaking with a person who has a lot of pain and stiffness, I'll say something like, "You should be a little better by tomorrow morning, a little less pain, a little more flexibility. You should be about 25% improved in a few days and probably close to 50% improved within ten days or so. How does that sound?" If I'm satisfied that the problem is a simple one, I'll say, "You'll probably experience a fair amount of relief by tomorrow morning." If the problem is simple and a lot was accomplished in the first treatment, I'll suggest that "You might even feel a little better right now. Let's take a look." And we'll evaluate the improvement and the amount of pain and/or reduced mobility that remains. I'll also comment that we'll reevaluate if we don't meet our expectations in a reasonable time frame. Or we will reevaluate if we've not obtained some good results in a few visits. I'll suggest a decision point where we might order x-rays if we haven't already done so, or note the circumstances in which an MRI or other special test would be useful.

A critical element in successful treatment outcomes is *communication*. I want my patient to know what's happening and where we're going every step of the way. I'm the doctor, of course, and you're seeking my expert

opinion, recommendations, and treatment. However, I request your coop-
eration and assistance in the process of getting you well. I'll outline an
approach, possibly share one or two elements in the decision-making
pathway, that is, how I arrived at these conclusions, and ask for your
agreement. Did I communicate effectively? Does this make sense to you?
Do you have any questions? Alternatively, not every person wants to know
everything. Perspective is helpful. Often just a few words are sufficient,
noting progress and steps for further improvement.

People who work out a lot want to get back to exercising, immediately.
Dancers need to get back to dance class, today if possible. Runners ask,
hopefully, "Can I run tomorrow morning?" Others say, "When can I go
back to the gym?" Well, being an athlete and not a very good patient, I am
acutely sensitive to these concerns. It would take a pretty major physical
problem for me to slow down or halt my activities, so I, too, want you to
get back ASAP. I see that as my primary function. I am not the doctor who
says, "stop doing that activity, you can't do that activity, find something a
little less strenuous". By now, people expect most of their doctors to say,
"Stop doing that." If that's my function, what good am I as a physician?
My job is to devise programs of recovery so that people can return to their
sports and exercises as quickly as possible.

My patients include championship ballroom dancers, mountain
climbers, marathon runners, 3-mile-a-day runners, masters tennis
competitors, tennis duffers, water skiers, motorcyclists, scratch golfers,
golfers who never break 100, rollerbladers, beach volleyball players, and
participants in water aerobics, step classes, and yoga classes. Are any of
them going to stop doing those things, simply because they hurt
themselves doing them? Not a chance. Do I want them to stop? No way.
I am fulfilling my end of the doctor-patient contract if I fix the person,
teach him how to function more efficiently and also avoid injury in the
future, and send him on his way, back to the wars.

Of course, all of this is in the context of an appropriate timeline. Rest is
key to recovery, so I emphasize avoiding the activity that recreates the

pain. However, rest does not necessarily mean sit around or lie down all day. Now, many neck and lower back injuries do need precisely this level of rest, for a few days. In such a case I explain that the early rest will enable the person to return to full function more quickly. Untimely early activity will most definitely cause setbacks and slow recovery. Occasionally the person learns this the hard way. Then we might have a conversation about *working hard* versus *overdoing it.*

It's a fine line. I was talking with Cathy the other day, a retired professional dancer who is now, after four years of study, a champion amateur ballroom dancer. Cathy has had one hip replaced and has pins and screws in her lower back following a three-level laminectomy. She is perfectly fit, an inspiring person. We met almost twenty years ago and I treat her occasionally for this or that. Recently, Cathy injured her lower back lifting weights and came to my office rather twisted and bent over, not walking very well. I determined that this was no more than it seemed, a simple soft-tissue injury, and treated her. As soon as she sat up, Cathy asked, "Can I rehearse tomorrow?" What's my answer? Now, I know her. Cathy's extraordinary, she's extraordinarily fit. *What would I do if it was me?* I find this an incredibly useful question.

If it was me, and I was rehearsing for something important, as she was now, I would work through the pain. I've done this many times in the past. On the other hand, I always need to remind myself that now I'm the *doctor,* and what's the best recommendation for my patient? In this case the answer was yes, go ahead and rehearse, and if it's no good we'll pick up the pieces tomorrow afternoon. The upside was she could rehearse; this was important and necessary, if possible. The downside was that she would be somewhat worse and we would have delayed recovery. Both she and I were willing to risk that, and the next day she was OK, a little better altogether.

Two days later, on Cathy's next visit, she was back to the beginning, fairly hobbling. What had happened? I suspected she had done too much, had *overdid it,* rather than gradually easing back into her routine. "Well," she said, "I think I hurt myself doing my abdominals." "OK," I said, thinking that probably wasn't all she did, "what else?" "Oh, I did a half-hour of swimming, went to dance class, lifted weights for an hour, then did stomach exercises." I laughed. She laughed, too, noticing that, yes, maybe she had worked too hard for someone recovering from a back sprain. We talked a little about that subtle difference, the distinction between working hard and doing too much. I spoke even though I knew I was preaching to the choir. She knows her body, it's a finely tuned instrument, and she will always push the limits, seeking new levels of excellence and performance.

In fact, this is what I want for all my patients. As a result, I will usually err on the side of activity rather than rest. I make this clear to people. I say, "I err on the side of activity. Sometimes that's not appropriate." And together we'll look, explore the alternatives, and reach a conclusion that will work for the person, provide the maximum benefit in terms of rest and activity, and get them well.

I had a recent example of this in my own training. I was running intervals, doing six quarter-miles at 2:05. The total run was five miles, including the run to the reservoir and back. Pretty normal stuff. After work on the following day I ran again, 3.5 miles around Central Park's lower loop. There are some nice uphill grades on this run, and recently I've been powering up the last two hills, at the end of the loop, running with some speed. One of them is a long, curving ascent, lasting for about one-quarter mile. It's great to be able to run up these hills, accelerating rather than slowing down, feeling strong rather than struggling. I ran out of the park and downhill from Fifth Avenue toward York Avenue.

On this night, two blocks before reaching my building, I felt a sudden, sharp pain in my left calf. Nothing unusual had happened. I hadn't tripped over a crack in the pavement or twisted to the side to avoid a leaping and snapping Jack Russell terrier, straining on its leash. Well, I've had pain before. Do I stop and walk the two blocks home? Right. I kept running, feeling that sharp pain with every push off and landing of that leg. This wasn't good and the pain persisted for two days.

Funny, I thought, I'm writing a book on being well and peak physical performance and here I am with a training injury of my own. How perfect. And, I thought, rats, my running has been going so well. I can't bear to miss several or more weeks of running to heal some stupid injury. I considered my alternatives, knowing I had to stop running for a while. I mean, it hurt to walk. So I applied the principle of relative rest. I went to the gym, replaced a few running sessions with weight-training, and rested my calf. On the fifth day I was pain-free and decided to lightly run two miles. I thought I'd run to the park, run a little inside the park, and run home.

Well, by the time I got to the park I felt so good that I ran the full lower loop and back. Oops. I thought, what if I was my patient and I reported this activity to myself on my next office visit? I shrugged my mental shoulders. It's a fine line between working hard and overdoing it. For my next few runs I took it easy, being careful, not pushing, very aware of sensations in the left calf. I ran the hills at a steady pace, not accelerating, just staying even, and had only a couple of twinges overall. I was fine and grateful that I had dodged a bullet. I might have needed to be off running for four weeks. The question remained, what had caused that calf strain?

I concluded that I "overdid it" rather than merely "worked hard". I hadn't rested sufficiently from my interval workout before running hard up the Central Park hills the next day. Had I done an easy, 3.5-mile run I might have avoided the calf strain. I acknowledge this is conjecture. I don't know what happened, but in most cases there's a cause related to an injury, and it's useful to determine that cause and learn from it. How do you know you're overdoing it? At the time, I didn't. Sometimes you only know in retrospect. Of course, "hindsight is 20/20". My next run after doing intervals will be easy, with minimal acceleration. A recovery run, really. I can self-correct from a training error, one that luckily didn't have too much of a consequence.

Should you be protective of yourself, very aware of the possibility of doing too much, afraid to challenge physical limits? No. One great goal of training and sports is to get better, to go beyond, to do more than you did the day before. Working hard can lead to injury; then you look for training errors and make modifications. And, possibly, you can catch yourself in the process of "overdoing" and say, "OK, tomorrow's another day. Time for a shower."

What is the context for training hard, reaching new milestones, pushing the envelope, and being consistently healthy and well? This is the crux of the matter, isn't it? The context is awareness, developing and causing a keen understanding of your physical capabilities and current limitations, and acting from, "What's *good* for me?" This is distinct from what my ego, wishes, desires, and fears might say I *should* be doing now. I remind myself that the times I've really hurt myself were when I either wasn't concentrating on what I was doing, that is, thinking of something else, or just showing off. You *do* know what's good for you, what's effective and appropriate during training, and you'll be doing that and not the other if you're present, listening and paying attention to your body's communication.

Now, returning to our doctor–patient interaction, at the conclusion of the first visit we've discussed the working diagnosis, possible further testing, methods of treatment, and the expected outcomes. Returning to exercise, as quickly as is feasible, is a critical outcome of treatment. *Relative rest* is a key concept in returning to previous levels of activity. Relative rest implies resting the injured part while continuing to exercise other muscle groups. For example, if I strained my calf running, I could continue to exercise by lifting weights—training my upper body, quadriceps and hamstrings. If I'm a tennis player and I've strained my rotator cuff or developed tendinitis in my elbow, I could continue to train by running or stair-climbing, and I could lift weights in a program specifically designed to recover from those types of injury. If I strained my pectoralis tendon doing dumbbell flyes, I could continue to lift weights, avoiding chest exercises until the tendon healed.

There's an interesting thing about relative rest. Remember when we were talking about cross-training, I said that combining training types provides dramatic gains in both areas being trained. If you're running and lifting weights, the running will make you stronger in the gym and the weight-training will make you faster on the track. Your muscles will get longer and you'll be more "ripped", with more muscular definition (more definition, *not* bulkier!) than if you were only doing one or the other. By now, this is well-known in sports communities. Swimmers lift weights. Basketball players lift weights. Ballet dancers lift weights. Weight-lifters run. Gymnasts run. Relative rest provides a similar cross-training effect: you'll likely come back stronger once the injury has healed because you've emphasized training other body parts, possibly training in a more complete fashion than prior to the injury. So I don't want my patients to rest. I want them to engage in *relative rest,* or *smart* rest. My questions are these: what can the person be doing and how soon can she be doing it?

OK. We've talked about my anticipated outcomes for patients. What are your anticipated outcomes of treatment? In my experience, most people want to be better *tomorrow!* And why not? Pain is unwelcome, uncomfortable, *annoying.* If the problem is spine-related, you experience pain on almost all types of motion, simply because the spine and its muscles are involved in all central body movements. So, please make the pain go away *now.* Well, my goal too is to make the pain go away as quickly as possible, and sometimes that means tomorrow or the next day. Most often, there is a longer time frame involved; my purpose is to shorten that time frame, do everything appropriate and necessary to achieve pain reduction and return to function. So on the next visit after the first treatment, and on each subsequent office visit, I'll ask, "How are you responding to treatment? What's better? How much better? What's not better?"

A person might respond, "I'm not better. I had less pain last night, I slept better, I'm a little more flexible this morning, *but it still hurts.*" This is a communication issue and I'll clarify my question and my intention in asking it. To me, "better" means "some improvement, some reduction, even temporarily, in either the intensity or frequency of the pain, or both". For the person, "better" means better, that is, *all* better. I'll explain that I'm looking for what was improved, even for a few hours. Did you sleep a little more comfortably? Was there a little less pain this morning? Is it a little easier to put on your shoes or socks? Was it less painful to get into and out of the taxicab? I'll emphasize that it's the improvement that counts, that if you were even a little improved then we're going in the right direction. I'll say that my question isn't, "Are you all better?", but rather, "Was there some noticeable improvement?" Over time, the small changes will add up to *all better.* That's where we intend to go. We'll get there with the degree of velocity that is possible given the particular circumstances. Again, people who are in good shape get better faster. Those who are deconditioned respond more slowly, in part because the recovery itself is a conditioning issue.

My patients participate in their treatment. It's a shared experience. It's a request on my part: I request that you help me help you get better. I have specific recommendations and a game plan, an outline of the progress anticipated in each case. I will provide specific treatment in my office and request that you follow my recommendations to facilitate your rehabilitation and recovery. These include postural corrections, stretching activities, and exercise. For most people, exercise can appropriately begin when the pain is two-thirds resolved. So another useful question I pose is, "If 100% is all better, how much better do you think you are?" I make this type of estimate for each person, and periodically I'll ask for the individual's subjective assessment, which provides critical information. It's a real-world check—does my estimation of what's going on match up with the patient's experience? Usually these two interpretations are pretty close. And, since we're looking for subjective milestones of 25% and 50% improvement, such a question provides the needed information.

We've talked about returning to exercise following injury. What about people who have never exercised with any consistency, or haven't done so for years? Let's say you're a person who doesn't exercise. First of all, it's not a black mark against you. You simply haven't exercised, that's all. I do suggest, however, that it's time to start, particularly if you're a patient in my office. The great thing about exercise is that you can begin any time and it's *always* beneficial. Of course, starting sooner is better than later, and best of all is starting *now.*

Let's talk about the person who is recovering from an injury and has not really exercised previously. You've hurt your neck or lower back, possibly had severe pain and loss of mobility, don't want to have that kind of experience again, and have a suspicion that exercise might be useful in preventing a recurrence. I ask about exercise when I take your history, possibly initiating or furthering an internal dialog you've been having on that very subject, something like, "if only I did some exercise, this wouldn't have happened", or "if I could lose some weight and do some exercise, I'd feel a whole lot better". Well, in a word, yes.

Stretching is the first component of any rehabilitative program. Hamstring and calf stretches can provide good relief for most mechanical lower back problems; quadriceps stretches are added as soon as possible. In fact, I recommend these lower extremity stretches for all persons who aren't exercising: simply, their muscles are tight and need to be lengthened on a consistent basis. Neck problems are also improved by doing leg stretches. Lower back muscles lengthen in response to decreasing torsion and torque on the pelvis. Neck muscles lengthen in response to decreasing stress from below. OK, you've been stretching for a week or two, it's going well, and you're making good improvement regarding your injury. What's next? Well, what would you like to do?

This is a key question. In my experience, no one is going to do what I *tell* them to do. A person might follow instructions for a while, but will probably give it up as soon as he leaves my sphere of influence (that is, treatment is completed). And since exercise wasn't a habit, in fact *not doing exercise* was the habit, the person will revert to old habits and stop doing the new stuff. This is all human and natural. A shift might occur if the person had a *choice* in the matter of exercising. So I give you a choice. I say something like, "Look, exercise is important in both the short-term and the long-term. Now, you don't have to do this. You're not a bad person if you don't. But my goal is to get you fixed as quickly as possible and prevent this kind of thing from happening in the future. If these are your goals, too, then exercise becomes a useful tool. And, who knows, it might even turn out to be fun." Something like that.

And then I say, "I'd like you to consider what kinds of exercise *you* might like to do, what you'd be willing to do. Let's talk about that when we see each other next." If I say, as the doctor, "you *should* start running" or "you *should* go to the gym and lift weights", there's not much freedom in that for you. It's not your choice. You might resist my recommendations altogether, or you might comply for a while because you want to be a good patient and you know you *should*, or you'll start the exercises and actually hurt yourself and have to stop, but that's OK because you really didn't want to anyway.

None of this stuff goes on if we have agreement, if the choice of exercise is your choice. So you go home and evaluate the options. I recommend running and weight-training as good possibilities, and I acknowledge that not everyone wants to do those things. Then we consider what you would like to do. We discuss the appropriateness, and possibly I'll make some specific other recommendation. Then we establish some guidelines for beginning and some near-term goals. And you start.

Now, for some people, walking is the best way to begin a training program. For example, you haven't exercised since high school and that was thirty years ago. Or you haven't exercised in ten years and you're fifty pounds overweight. Nothing is wrong, those are simply the facts, and it's just not appropriate to begin anything more rigorous than walking. Walking will provide a foundation upon which we can build. Remember, the great benefit of exercise is that you can always start right here, right now.

A person might say, "But I already walk. I walk a lot." Well, there are a few differences between walking for exercise and walking to work or to the store. Both the intention and the circumstances are different. When you walk for exercise, you're specifically doing *that*. You've set aside time for this activity. You've stretched beforehand. You're wearing workout-type clothes. And you have the intention of *walking*. You might finish by arriving at your office, showering and changing there. Or you might finish your walk at the supermarket, and do your shopping. However, the walking part of your trip was a specific activity unto itself—it was designed to be *exercise*.

How to begin? First, I recommend buying a runner's watch. This watch can also be used for measuring elapsed time (the "chronometer" setting). If you haven't done much walking in a while, start with a medium-paced twelve minute walk. You don't want to struggle here, you just want to walk for twelve minutes. Set your chronometer for six minutes and place it in the repeat mode. Push the button and go. After six minutes your watch will beep, signaling you to turn around and head back home. With the intention of walking four or five times a week, do another twelve minutes tomorrow, and add a minute to your routine every few days or so, building up comfortably to a thirty-minute medium-paced walk. Having reached this goal, now you can begin *brisk* walking.

Walking is good exercise and brisk walking is even better. Start with brisk walking for fifteen minutes, building up gradually to forty minutes or more. In brisk walking you are *moving:* moving quickly, arms and legs thrusting forward and back easily, in purposeful opposition. Brisk walking is a natural, graceful accentuation of the movements utilized in casual walking. Your limb actions are in control, not flailing, but the velocity is increased and the stride is lengthened. Increase your speed gradually, from workout to workout, building in intensity from modest to brisk. Also, gently increase the speed within the workout itself. Within eight weeks (remember we started basically from ground zero) you have advanced to a rigorous workout program, forty or more minutes of brisk walking, which you do four or so times per week. You're perspiring after your workout, you've gotten past the huffing and puffing stage, and you're beginning to feel *very good* about yourself. And, remarkably, you've begun to lose weight!

Let's talk about the *target zone* for efficient cardiovascular exercise. The target zone refers to how hard your heart is working during exercise, that is, how many times your heart beats per minute. It's a simple, straightforward parameter: too fast is inefficient in terms of overwork and is potentially harmful; too slow is not working hard enough to derive a cardiovascular benefit, that is, you're wasting your time. Target zones are easily calculated: subtract your age from 220; multiply this result by both 60% and 80%. These two results represent the range of values that is your target zone. For example, if you are 40 years old, then

$$220-40 = 180; 180 \text{ X } 0.60 = 108$$
$$220-40 = 180; 180 \text{ X } 0.80 = 144$$

For a 40-year-old, the target zone for efficient cardiovascular exercise is 108–144 beats per minute. How do you utilize this number in practice? To determine how fast your heart is beating during exercise, stop for a moment and take your pulse for ten seconds. Ten seconds, of course, is one-sixth of a minute. The target zone of 108–144 beats per minute is the same as a range of 18–24 beats every ten seconds. So, if you're 40 years old, you know you're training efficiently if you count between 18 and 24 beats in a ten-second interval. Now go back to your training. If you were under 18 heartbeats in ten seconds, work a little harder; if you were over 24, slow down a little.

Here are target zone ranges for a number of age groups:

- Age 30: 19–25 beats in ten seconds
- Age 40: 18–24
- Age 50: 17–23
- Age 60: 16–21

- Age 70: 15–20
- Age 80: 14–19

You don't have to be a fanatic about this. Rather, the target zone information provides a background of both effectiveness and safety. When you are comfortably along in your training, target zone calculations are no longer needed.

OK. We've looked extensively at the nature of the doctor–patient interaction when you go to a chiropractor's office for the first time. At the conclusion of the first visit, after taking a history and performing an orthopedic/neurologic/biomechanical examination, your chiropractor will review the working diagnosis, possible additional tests, methods of treatment, and anticipated outcomes. He will probably suggest that an exercise program will be an important part of recovery. Specific discussions about exercise could begin after a person is about 50% improved. You receive treatment, do your stretches and exercises, get better, and are discharged.

How do you choose the type of specialist you will see? Medicine is empiric, that is, the usefulness of a treatment is evaluated based on the response to that treatment. If it works, keep going; if not, initiate a different method of therapy. The bottom line is—whatever works, works. There is no intrinsic goodness in one type of treatment versus another. Medication, manipulation, and physical therapy are all valid and useful methods. For some cases, all three approaches are needed. For others, one method is sufficient. One criterion for selection could be efficiency: how quickly does the particular specialist achieve very good to excellent results? Word of mouth is helpful. Do you know someone who had a similar injury and was very satisfied with his treatment?

Other criteria include the location and severity of the injury. The vast majority of spine-related problems can be treated effectively by a chiropractor—she is the specialist who treats spine cases all day long. Severe spinal pain is best treated initially with medication. Chiropractic manipulation may be useful in the secondary phase of treatment; physical therapy may be a third treatment phase. Injuries to the extremities are best handled by physicians specializing in treatment of sports-related conditions. Such a doctor, whether a chiropractor, orthopedic surgeon, or physiatrist, has been *specifically* trained to treat sports-related conditions, and has special expertise in the areas of biomechanics and rehabilitation. Severe injuries should be evaluated by an orthopedic surgeon. In general, the vast majority of injuries are not severe and may be seen by a chiropractor or physiatrist. Physical therapists may be utilized in the latter stages of treatment for any sports-type injury.

What style of treatment are you comfortable with? For me, I would like to know that my doctor explored the alternatives and developed a treatment plan that was *right for me,* not one that was based on a preconceived set of ideas or rigid hypotheses. A lot of methods "work". My only concern is, will this method work for me? Will I recover in a reasonable period of time and is there the possibility that I will come back stronger? Does my doctor encourage *active care,* that is, does she offer mechanisms by which I can help her help me now, and help myself in the future? These are some areas that can help determine whether "I'm in the right place".

Now let's discuss plans and programs for recovering from the typical training injuries that may occur from time to time. Our goals always are (1) make a specific and accurate diagnosis, (2) design and implement a realistic and attainable rehabilitation program that a person can maintain *on his or her own,* and (3) help the patient *come back stronger.*

---▼---

CHAPTER 10

COMING BACK STRONGER: INJURY AS OPPORTUNITY

I've had my share of injuries. It's a long list: hamstring tears, ankle sprains, rotator cuff strains, finger sprains, elbow strains, shin splints, you name it. I'm not complaining. I've learned something important from most of these injuries and been able to apply that knowledge to the treatment of patients. And, those breakdowns have provided the context for me to be able to write this book! If you play hard, doing physical stuff, injuries are a fact of life. Of course, you'll have many more injuries if you don't train and prepare effectively and if your technique is sloppy. But, even with the best training, injuries will come. Now, having sustained an injury, what are you going to do?

Well, you might start by seeing a sports doctor (chiropractor, physiatrist, or orthopedic surgeon—one who *specializes* in the treatment of sports-related injuries). However, if you are like me, you probably won't do that. I'd much rather fix something on my own, or wait it out and expect to get better with time. The catch, of course, the *difference,* is that I'm a sports doc myself. I treat these conditions, and expect that I can pretty well handle my own injuries. In this chapter we'll discuss techniques on managing injuries and how to rehabilitate yourself so that you come back both *quicker* and *stronger.* Please note this is not a chapter on medical treatment and is not meant to substitute for such treatment. My intent is to present information and instruction on rehabilitation: things you can do to help yourself get back to doing the activities you want to do.

Most sports-type injuries affect one of the following structures: shoulder, elbow, wrist, knee, ankle, and spine. Shoulder injuries typically involve the rotator cuff; less commonly, the origin of the biceps muscle may be affected. Elbow injuries are often described as "tennis elbow": this pain on the outside of the elbow may or may not be caused by playing tennis. Elbow injury may also occur to the inside of the elbow (historically known as "golfer's elbow"). Wrist and ankle injuries may involve strains (muscles), sprains (ligaments), or combined muscle/ligament injuries. Knee sprains may involve the ligaments and/or menisci (knee cartilage). There may be acute strains around the knee, involving the hamstring or quadriceps tendons, and also vague, achy/sharp, generalized pain involving one or both knees. We'll evaluate each of these conditions in some detail.

Again, when is it appropriate to seek professional advice? Here are good basic guidelines. If you've suffered an acute injury and there is pain when you're at rest, in other words, when you're sitting or lying down, you probably should be examined by a physician. If your pain is severe, you should be examined by a physician. If you have *any* suspicion that you might have sustained a fracture, you should be examined by a physician. Or, if you've sustained an acute injury but are not in any of the above categories, and the pain lasts for more than 72 hours, you should be examined by a physician. For pain that is slowly developing (commonly representing an overuse condition), the first criterion is applicable: if pain is now present at rest, you should be examined by a physician. We've just described the minority of problems, the ones that need a doctor's immediate attention. Our discussion here concerning rehabilitation relates to the majority of conditions: acute injuries that are mild-to-moderate and chronic problems due to repetition/overuse and faulty biomechanics.

Rotator Cuffs

Let's look at shoulder problems first. These injuries might involve the rotator cuff, a musculotendinous hood comprised of four individual muscles. The rotator cuff covers many structures: the joint between the humerus and scapula (arm bone and shoulder blade); the deltoid muscle, located on the upper and outer part of the arm; the origin of the biceps muscle; and the shoulder joint itself. Golf, tennis, baseball, rowing, weight-training, dancing, and skiing are examples of activities that might, over time, lead to a shoulder injury. In the mid-1980s, during the high-impact aerobics boom, I suffered a bad rotator cuff strain in one of those classes. High-impact aerobics was a lot of fun, but people had a *lot* of injuries. Or, of course, you could simply reach up to get something off a top shelf, and strain your rotator cuff, biceps, or deltoid.

What is the rotator cuff and what does it do? The rotator cuff is composed of four individual muscles: (1) the subscapularis, located on the front of the scapula; (2) the supraspinatus, located on the back of the scapula, above its horizontal bony ridge; (3) the infraspinatus, located on the back of the scapula, below its horizontal bony ridge; and (4) the teres minor, a smaller muscle located on the back and side of the scapula. The subscapularis rotates the arm inward; the supraspinatus lifts the arm to the side; and the infraspinatus and teres minor rotate the arm outward. Each muscle inserts on and around the head of the humerus, crossing over the arm–scapula joint (glenohumeral joint), and together these musculotendinous insertions form a hood or "cuff" over the glenohumeral joint. Thus, the "rotator cuff", whose function is to elevate the arm to the side and turn it in and out. It's easy to see how optimal rotator cuff function would be critical to a baseball pitcher, for example, or a tennis player or ballet dancer, or a normally functioning human being.

Injuries of the rotator cuff are common, and part of the failure is inherent in the design. The shoulder joint has the greatest mobility of any joint in the body: it can rotate through a 360° arc of motion in two planes. Stability is sacrificed for this extreme mobility. For example, the shoulder is the most commonly dislocated joint: shoulder dislocations comprise about 50% of all dislocations. So the rotator cuff tendon is placed under significant tensile forces during normal activity. And, interestingly, part of its blood supply undergoes a pulleying type of traction during full elevation to the side (this movement is called *abduction*). Thus, any time the arm is fully abducted, a region of the rotator cuff is experiencing a temporary decrease in or loss of blood supply.

This region has been called the *critical zone* and it is a typical site for rotator cuff failure. Additionally, the rotator cuff tendon may become frayed and worn over time due to its constant contact with the bony prominences that comprise the shoulder joint. A degenerative syndrome of the shoulder may involve the joint itself, the acromion process (a flange of bone extending from the shoulder blade, arching over the shoulder "socket"), the rotator cuff tendon, and the tendon forming the origin of the biceps. So there is the possibility of a number of regional shoulder problems.

What are some of the symptoms of a rotator cuff injury? Painful and restricted ranges of motion of the shoulder is the primary symptom of an impaired rotator cuff. Raising the arm to the side and up, raising the arm forward and up, and/or turning the arm in or out may all reproduce shoulder pain. It hurts to brush your hair, it hurts to place something on an overhead shelf, it hurts to throw a ball, it hurts to swing your arm in aerobics class. Other symptoms include stiffness of the shoulder, limitation of motion, and weakness. Of course, this all sounds pretty bad, but problems range from mild to severe, severe representing rupture of the rotator cuff tendon, probably necessitating surgery. We are concerned here with mild to moderate rotator cuff injuries, which can be rehabilitated conservatively (conservatively means without surgery).

Thus, there are inherent structural weaknesses of the shoulder, related to its great flexibility and mobility. I'm not suggesting the shoulder is *weak,* but rather it is more likely to be injured than, say, your hip or your finger. Weight-training is the best method for strengthening the shoulder, increasing local blood supply by causing more capillaries to be built, and thus decreasing the local susceptibility to injury. Logically, weight-training is a great tool in rehabilitation from any injury, but you have to build up to it—weight-training is a later stage of rehabilitation. The first stage in managing a rotator cuff injury is restoring mobility, that is, improving ranges of motion.

OK. You've acutely injured your shoulder, either by killer-serving a tennis ball or by putting your hat on the top shelf of your closet, and you have shoulder pain, stiffness, limited mobility, and/or weakness. Or, possibly, these things have developed over time and you're not getting better but, rather, worsening. You see your sports physician-of-choice and learn you have a rotator cuff injury (probably termed a *strain*—remember, a strain is an injury to a muscle–tendon unit). Here are a number of things you can do to restore mobility, increase strength, get better faster, and *stay* better.

The first few things are simple, and it will feel like you aren't really doing much of anything. That's the idea. Basic movements restore ranges of motion. In the early part of recovery from any injury, acute or chronic, there should be no *effort,* no *stress.* The first rehabilitative activity is termed *finger-walking.* Stand about 18 inches away from a wall, positioned so that your torso is perpendicular to the wall. Reach your arm out to the side and touch the wall with the tips of your fingers. There should be a slight elbow bend, about 30 degrees or so (Figure 10.1).

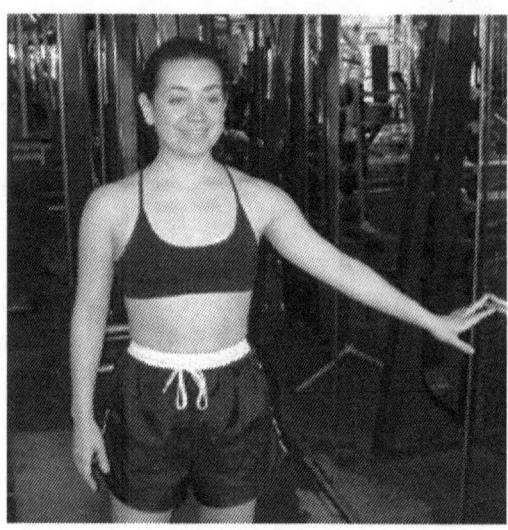

Figure 10.1

If your arm is straight, you're too far away from the wall. In this starting position your hand and fingers are at about shoulder height (we'll call this 90°of abduction—0 degrees of abduction is when your arm is hanging at your side; 180° is when your arm is lifted straight overhead).

Slowly walk your fingers up the wall as high as you can go (Figure 10.2). At maximum height you might reach 160° of abduction. Walk your fingers slowly all the way down the wall and then repeat, walking your fingers up the wall as high as you can go. Do the activity ten times. Don't force anything: shoulder pain means that's as high as you can go. Don't go higher than the position that creates pain.

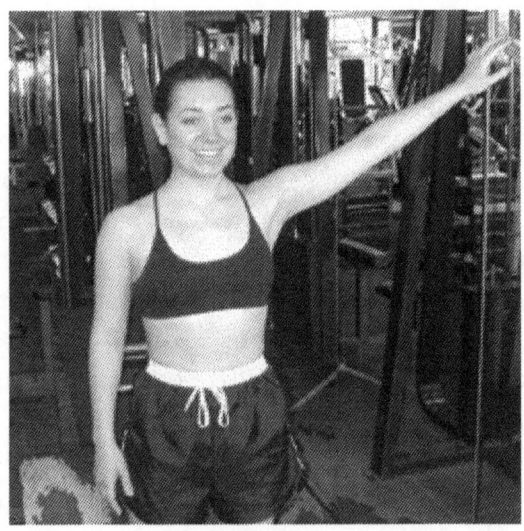

Figure 10.2

Next, face the wall, standing about 18 inches away, extend your arm, and place your fingers on the wall. Walk your fingers up the wall, as high as you can go, and slowly walk your fingers all the way down the wall. This movement is called forward flexion. Do this ten times. If your shoulder injury is more severe, you might need to start at a lower elevation than 90° of abduction or forward flexion. Start where you can and do the finger-walking as high as you can, not exceeding the point of pain. As you continue the exercise over days and weeks, your range of motion will improve. Finger-walking is a classical rehabilitative activity for improving shoulder ranges of motion.

The next basic, simple activity is the *pendulum* exercise. Let's say the right shoulder is the one being rehabilitated. Sit at the edge of a hard chair and bend your torso forward. Support your weight by activating your stomach muscles and resting your left hand on your right knee and your left forearm on your left inner thigh. Let your right arm dangle to the side and, slowly and gently, begin to swing the arm in a small circle, the movement being initiated by a gentle swaying of your torso. Slowly increase the diameter of the circle, from a beginning of about six inches to a maximum of about 18 inches. The whole routine should take about a minute.

Do both activities, finger-walking and the pendulum, several times each day. When full, painless ranges of motion are restored it's time to begin the next phase of rehabilitation: resisted ranges of motion. Resisted ranges of motion uses *surgical tubing* to provide the resistance. Surgical tubing is inexpensive and available from any surgical supply store. Cut a four-foot (if you're about six feet tall) or 3.5-foot (if you're closer to five-and-a-half feet tall) length of tubing. Place one end of it under your foot (step on it firmly so that a few inches of tubing extends past the side of your foot; you don't want the tubing to snap up while you are doing the exercise). Wrap the other end of the surgical tubing around your hand, maintaining a good grip.

Starting with your arm at your side and your palm facing down, raise your arm forward and up. You're not going too far, maybe six to ten inches or so, depending on how much slack there is in the tubing. There should be no straining, just meet the resistance provided by the tubing and go as far as you can, maintaining the limit of the stretch for several seconds (Figure 10.3). Rest a moment and repeat, for a total of six repetitions. The tubing allows you to work your shoulder muscles within a narrowly defined, protected limit. This method is similar to isometric exercise—it's not formally isometric because there is a little movement involved.

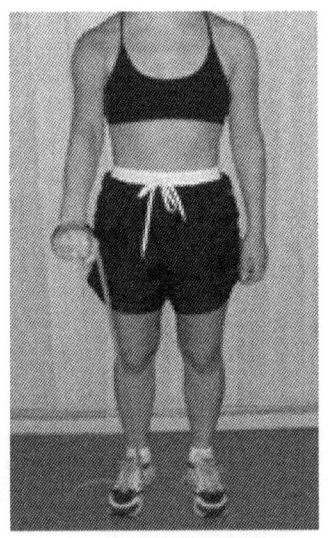 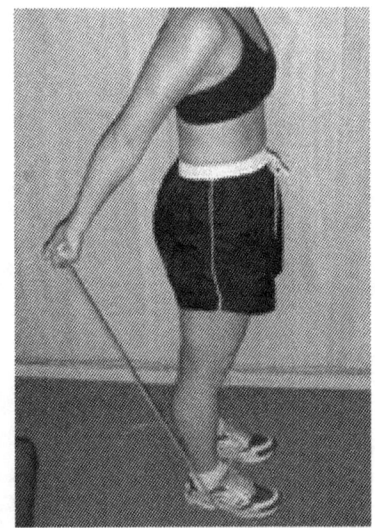

Figure 10.3 **Figure 10.4**

You just did *forward flexion*. Now, from the same starting position, bring the arm straight back as far as you can, maintain the stretch for several seconds, and relax (Figure 10.4). Do six repetitions total. This exercise strengthens your shoulder in *extension*.

Next, from the initial position, lift your arm to the side and up, as far as you can go (Figure 10.5). Hold, relax, repeat. This is *abduction*. Next, from the initial position, bring your arm in the opposite direction, that is, straight across your body moving from right to left (Figure 10.6). You're not going too far here—you might get as far as the outside of your left thigh. This movement is *adduction*—the normal range of motion for adduction is about one-third of that for abduction.

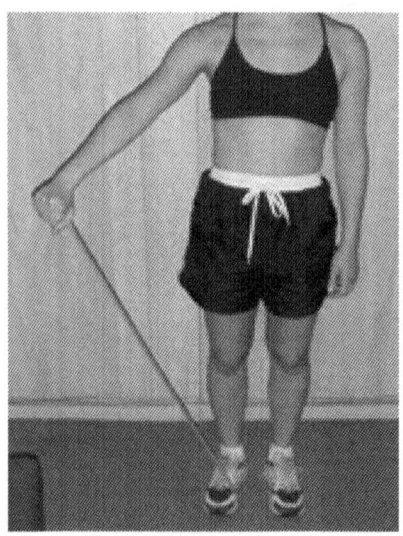 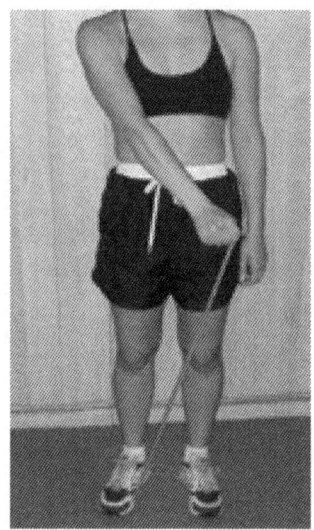

Figure 10.5   **Figure 10.6**

Next, we'll do external and internal rotation. The setup is a little more complex. Close a door and wrap one end of the tubing around the doorknob. Make sure it is secure, so it does not fly off when you're doing the exercise. Stand with your left side facing the doorknob (your torso is at a right angle to the door frame). Wrap the other end of the tubing around your right hand (start from the middle of the tubing, so there's not so much slack). With your right arm at your side and your right elbow bent to a 90° angle, move your right forearm and hand away from your body while keeping your elbow at your side (Figure 10.7). This movement is *external rotation*. Hold, relax, repeat. Do six repetitions total. Next, turn around so your right side is facing the doorknob (your torso is at a right angle to the door frame). Wrap the tubing around your right hand, leaving some slack. Using the same starting position as that for external rotation, move your right forearm and hand across the center of your body, moving from right to left (Figure 10.8). You're only able to move a very short distance here, maybe 20° in total. This is *internal rotation*. Again, do six repetitions.

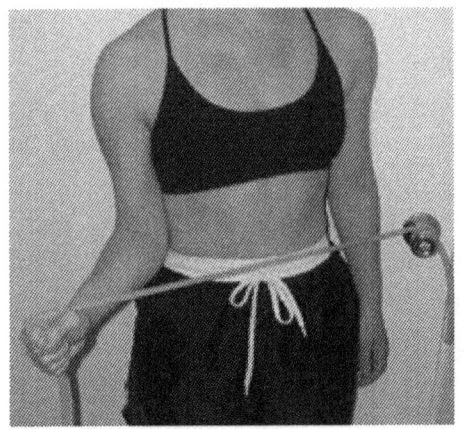

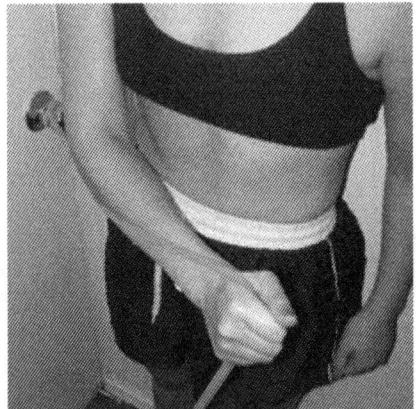

Figure 10.7   **Figure 10.8**

Congratulations! You've just done a complete isometric routine for your rotator cuff. Supporting muscles, such as the deltoid, latissimus, and trapezius, have also been trained. Do this routine five times per week for several weeks, building up to eight reps in each direction. Over time, these exercises will improve painless ranges of motion and increase strength of the shoulder girdle. When painless mobility has been restored, you can begin shoulder exercises with weights.

The surgical tubing routines are isometric. Exercises using free weights or weight machines are *resistive*, that is, you move a weight through a plane of motion. In Chapter 6 we described a routine of four exercises for the shoulder: military press, upright row, lateral raise, and bent-over raise. Military press is a compound shoulder exercise, training all three sections of the deltoid. The upright row specifically trains the anterior deltoid; the lateral raise trains the middle deltoid; and the bent-over raise trains the posterior deltoid. These exercises involve the rotator cuff as secondary supports: the supraspinatus participates in the lateral raise, the teres minor and infraspinatus function in the bent-over raise. To rehabilitate a rotator cuff injury we'll utilize the four basic shoulder exercises and add one specifically designed to train the shoulder rotators.

In this exercise you lie on a flat bench with your heels up on the end of the bench and your knees bent at a 90° angle. Let's continue to rehabilitate a right rotator cuff injury. Hold a light dumbbell in your right hand, with your elbow bent at a 90° angle and touching your right side. Keeping your elbow at your side and maintaining the 90° elbow bend, rotate your right arm outward so the weight moves away from your body. This is the starting position (Figure 10.9). One repetition involves rotating your arm inward so the weight moves across your body (Figure 10.10), and then rotating your arm outward so the weight moves back across your body to the starting position. The total normal arc of motion, combining both internal and external rotation, is about 120°.

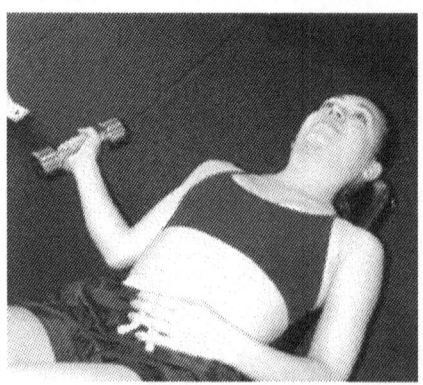
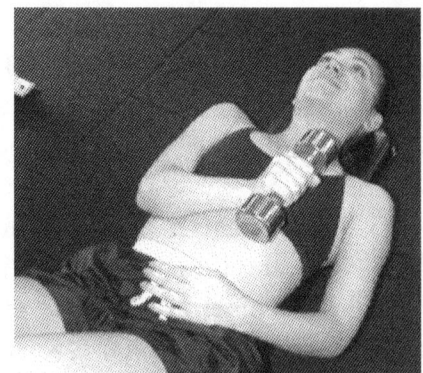

Figure 10.9   Figure 10.10

The goal is to build up to three sets of ten to twelve reps for each of the five exercises. Rehabilitation necessarily uses light weights. If you've never lifted weights before, use a five-pound dumbbell for the military presses, upright rows, and lateral raises. Use a three-pounder for the bent-over raises and the flat rotation exercise. If you've already been weight-training consistently, start with ten-pounders for the first three exercises and eight-pounders for the bent-over raise and flat rotations. Eight-pound dumbbells? Yes. Heavier is definitely *not* better in rehabilitation. Start light and build back up over several weeks. If there is any shoulder pain at all you are working too heavy: drop the weight to the next lighter dumbbell. Start light and do three sets of six to eight reps. Build to three sets of twelve over a number of sessions. Then go to the next heavier pair of dumbbells and do three sets of eight, building up weight and reps in this sequence.

You can discontinue finger-walking and the pendulum movement when you have full and painless forward flexion and abduction (about 180° each). You can move from surgical tubing isometrics to weight-training when you're strong enough to do three sets of eight reps in each of the six directions of motion. Once you've begun lifting weights you can attempt to return to a sporting activity. If you're going back to tennis, work on your ground strokes for a while. Get your swing back, and after a few sessions, do some easy serving. Same thing for golf. Work on your swing. The length on your drive will come back over time. Everything's a process. Come back slowly and you will come back stronger.

Tennis Elbow

What about elbow problems, particularly *tennis elbow?* Tennis elbow refers to pain over and around the small bony protuberance on the outside of the elbow. There can also be pain in a similar location on the *inside* of the elbow, historically known as *golfer's elbow.* These two pain syndromes can be considered as one problem and addressed similarly. Whichever one develops depends on the type and direction of repetitive mechanical stress placed on the elbow. Tennis elbow, known as *lateral epicondylitis* (the small bony protuberances are the *epicondyles*), is an injury to the origin of the muscle group that extends the wrist (lifts the hand up if the palm is oriented downward). These muscles also perform the function of *supination*, that is, rotating the forearm so the forearm and palm face up.

The extensor-supinator muscles originate on the lateral epicondyle, a small projection of bone on the bottom of the humerus. The origin is broad, with only a minimal blood supply.

The muscle group that originates on the inside of the elbow, on the *medial epicondyle,* flexes the wrist (lifts the hand up if the palm is oriented upward) and pronates the forearm (rotates the forearm so the forearm and palm face down). The flexor-pronator origin is similarly broad with a tenuous blood supply. Musculotendinous strains tend to heal slowly and with difficulty because of the limited blood supply in the region of the elbow.

Thus, as a result of the structural design, elbow strains tend to linger. Healing is slow because of the lack of sufficient oxygen and other nutrients. What to do? We'll look at brand new, acute elbow injuries, and then we'll discuss management of those nagging, chronic elbow strains. I'll start by saying that any elbow pain must be treated with caution and respect. The concern is that the sudden, sharp elbow pain you experience today may, if ignored, progress to a long-term, nonresolving, activity-limiting problem. I'm not suggesting that you be an alarmist. Anybody can have a little elbow twinge. However, a number of little twinges over a few training sessions is a problem, and a one-time intense, searing pain is a definite concern.

We're going to digress for a moment and discuss general methods for home treatment of many acute injuries. First, of course, cease the activity that caused the pain. Pain implies tearing, at least on the microscopic level, of muscle fibers around the injured joint, with associated disruption of tiny capillaries. Treatment of mild to moderate acute injuries is fairly standard and typical. These injuries do not involve total disruption of tendons or ligaments and can be treated conservatively, that is, without the need for surgical repair. Acute care includes rest, ice, compression, and elevation, these methods forming the mnemonic, *RICE.* Rest may imply complete rest of the injured part, or it may mean *relative rest,* that is, avoiding activities that cause pain. Elevation is appropriate for lower extremity injuries such as ankle sprains that involve a fair amount of tissue swelling. Compression may be indicated, particularly for injuries that have produced swelling.

Ice is a useful method for treating acute injuries. Many people, including a number of physicians, are unclear about the indications for applying ice versus heat. Briefly, you can never go wrong by applying ice, whereas you can have some bad consequences by applying heat inappropriately. Generally, ice is utilized for acute injuries within a 72-hour time frame from the onset of the injury. Some sources recommend that ice be used within the first 48 hours—in most cases, ice is effective for up to 72 hours following an injury.

Ice has several physiologic effects which make it useful in the acute setting. The application of ice constricts local small blood vessels, reducing local swelling. Acute injury disrupts capillaries, causing blood to leak into the tissue spaces, where it doesn't belong. This uncontained blood creates pressure on nerve endings, causing pain. Pressure is also placed on other cells and tissues, causing injury and possibly cell death. Thus, it's important to limit the amount of blood leaking out of injured capillaries. Ice performs this function. Ice also slows the transmission of nerve impulses, reducing pain and creating a sedative effect. Therefore, ice reduces swelling, reduces pain, and is a sedative.

The most important thing to remember when applying ice is to avoid damaging the skin. Ice packs are always wrapped in a towel; ice is almost never applied directly to the skin. How long should ice be applied? There's no firm rule here. I recommend that an ice pack be applied for 15 minutes every two hours for a moderate acute injury. If the injury is mild, ice can be applied for 15 minutes every three hours or so. A minimum of two or three applications per day is recommended. It's not necessary to be obsessive about applying ice; you'll know instinctively when it's time to reapply the cold. Ice packs are useful for all types of acute injuries. An injured joint can be wrapped in ice, for example, for the allotted time period. Another form of ice therapy is the *ice massage.*

Ice massage is used for injuries to long muscles, for example, the quadriceps and hamstring groups, or upper and lower back musculature. You'll freeze water in a paper cup and then remove the top half-inch of the cup with a knife. Now you have an exposed ice surface with a type of handle. Apply the ice directly to the skin and rub it along the injured muscle, longitudinally, going up and down slowly for *no more* than 5 minutes. Ice massage feels great and is relaxing and soothing, but *do not* exceed 5 minutes at a time. Ice massage can be repeated every hour or so, for up to five applications a day.

Back to specifics. *Compression* for relief of tennis elbow symptoms is provided by a two-inch-thick elastic support that has a Velcro closure. The support is applied so that its top edge is about 1.5 inches below the elbow. The support effectively shortens the origin of the affected muscle group— the contraction of the muscle does not reach the irritated tissues around the elbow itself. The support provides rest for the injured muscle fibers at the origin, allowing for faster healing. The brace can be worn all day.

Rehabilitative exercises can begin when the acute pain of the elbow injury has subsided and you can shake a person's hand with only minimal pain. As usual, these exercises are easy and basic. They are designed to increase the strength of the wrist extensors and flexors, which originate, respectively, on the outer and inner aspects of the elbow joint. Additionally, exercising these muscle groups will improve circulation to the elbow, adding capillaries and increasing the local blood supply. Very light dumbbells are used initially, three-pounders for women and possibly five-pounders for men. Don't be embarrassed to use a very light weight in the beginning. There should be *no* pain during any rehabilitative exercise. Pain implies either that you're not ready to do the exercise, or you're ready but are using too much weight.

Elbow rehabilitation involves three exercises: wrist flexion, wrist extension, and pronation/supination. The exercises are done in a seated position; the elbow is bent at 30–45° throughout. For wrist flexion, the palm faces upward. Grasp a dumbbell with your wrist in a neutral position

(Figure 10.11). Flex the wrist, so that the palm elevates. Go to a position of full wrist flexion, without straining (Figure 10.12). Relax and allow the wrist to return to the starting position. Start with eight repetitions.

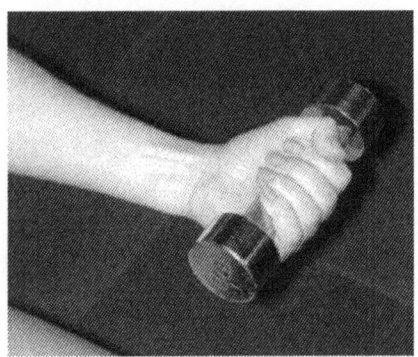
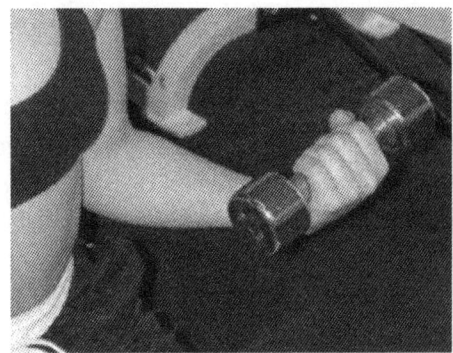

Figure 10.11   Figure10.12

Then turn the wrist over so that the palm faces downward (Figure 10.13). (This motion is termed *pronation.*) Wrist extension is accomplished by raising the wrist as high as it will go, without straining (Figure 10.14). Relax and return the wrist to a neutral position. Do eight repetitions.

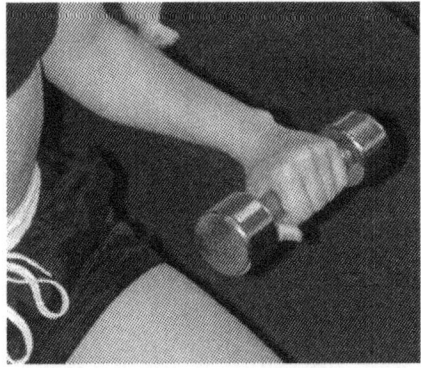
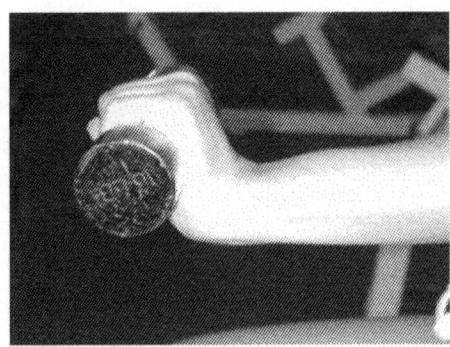

Figure 10.13   Figure 10.14

Next, starting with the palm facing upward, turn the palm downward (pronation) and return the palm to an upward position (supination). This is one repetition of the pronation/supination exercise. Do eight repetitions. Three exercises, eight repetitions each, will constitute one set of elbow rehab. Do a set with the noninjured arm. Do three sets total for each arm.

Do these exercises four or five times a week, building up to three sets of twelve repetitions. If you feel pain, you're doing too much, and drop the reps or lower the weight. Once you're doing three sets of twelve, increase the weight and start over with eight reps. If you were using a three-pound dumbbell, go up to a five-pounder. If you were using a five-pounder, go up to an eight-pound dumbbell.

When can you go back to your sport? When you can shake somebody's hand without experiencing elbow pain, you have recovered pretty well and may begin hitting some tennis balls or going to the driving range. Return to activity slowly, and ice your elbow afterward as a precaution (one 15-minute application of an ice pack should be sufficient) for the first two weeks. Consider whether you have a mechanical flaw that possibly created the elbow strain. Would tennis or golf lessons be helpful? Probably. Your mechanics are rusty anyway from inaction and instruction can provide inspiration as well as technique. After about twelve weeks you can discontinue the program of elbow weight-training; however, doing these exercises once a week or so may still be beneficial.

I've described rehabilitation of an acute elbow injury, in which full recovery from moderate injury can be expected. However, left *untreated*, elbow strains tend not to resolve, but rather, tend to become chronic. Chronic, untreated elbow pain of more than three months duration is notoriously difficult to remedy. Such a problem certainly requires a physician's attention. Methods employed may include friction massage, trigger point release, ultrasound, or even cortisone injection. Response is slow and uncertain. It's best to have acute elbow injuries evaluated immediately and begin rehabilitation as soon as possible.

Knee Injuries

Knee injuries may be acute and sudden or chronic and slowly developing. Everyone knows about "ACL tears" and "MCL tears", referring, respectively, to severe injuries of the anterior cruciate and medial collateral ligaments. I've heard conversations about these injuries in the elevator of my apartment building. In the past, a ruptured ACL meant the end of a career for a professional athlete. However, within the last ten years, startling advances in surgical technique and graft management have enabled athletes to return to professional sports within a year, and sometimes sooner.

These powerful and successful procedures are likewise available to homemakers and stockbrokers, since severe knee derangement can occur while skiing or rollerblading, playing playground football or basketball, or from slipping on ice. For the most part, it's obvious when a person tears his MCL and/or ACL. The sudden tearing of the ligament makes a *popping* sound; you hear a "pop". There is significant pain and, usually, a fair amount of swelling within the first twenty-four hours. Magnetic resonance imaging, which shows the body's internal architecture in three dimensions, has great diagnostic accuracy in evaluating MCL and ACL injuries.

Severe knee problems are correctly handled by an orthopedic surgeon. We'll discuss more commonly experienced, mild to moderate knee pain that is nonspecific in nature, that is, not produced by an acute traumatic injury. The type of pain I'm describing is an achiness or soreness, possibly sharp at times, experienced *around* the knee joint. The pain might variously be on the inside of the patella (kneecap), on the outside of the patella, underneath it, or at all three locations simultaneously. Thus, this type of pain is migratory and generalized. Frequently, the pain is present in *both* knees. The knee *hurts*. Your knee doesn't feel *normal*.

There are a number of physical problems associated with this type of knee pain. Often, there will be knee pain climbing and/or going down stairs. Repeated flexing and extending the knee, as in walking or running, will create knee pain. Characteristically, the knee will *give way,* or buckle, when standing in one place for a period of time, for example, when washing dishes or waiting for a bus. There may be grating or grinding sounds in the knee. Over time, the problem is probably worsening. There is usually no history of an acute knee injury—the knee problem began without cause.

Generalized, nonspecific knee pain has been notoriously difficult to treat. Up until the last several years, people with nontraumatic knee pain were diagnosed as having "chondromalacia", a term that describes softening of the cartilage lining the undersurface of the patella. Surgery was even performed, utilizing an arthroscope to scrape off the presumably problematic degenerated cartilage. Mostly, these procedures were ineffective. Of course, surgery was recommended when conservative treatment had failed, but a fair conclusion is that the conservative approaches were poorly designed because the underlying problem was not well understood.

One principle of rehabilitation is to build up the surrounding musculature to support a weakened or damaged joint. Earlier we talked about strengthening the rotator cuff to support shoulder mechanics. The knee is made up of the lower end of the thigh bone, the upper end of the shin bone, the patella, and the muscles, tendons, ligaments, and cartilage that hold these bones together. The patella itself is contained within the quadriceps tendon. It was logical to conclude that building up the quadriceps would be helpful in cases of diffuse knee pain.

People were instructed to do "quad sets", a series of leg extensions utilizing a weight machine or weights attached to the person's ankle. I remember doing these quad sets, thirty years ago, sitting on a table at home with a bag containing a couple of cans of soup swinging from my ankle. The weight attachments became more sophisticated over the next fifteen years, but the results were the same.

Basically, this approach never worked, and a lot of people had their knees "scoped" with no postsurgical benefit. Current methods of rehabilitating diffuse knee pain are based on sports medicine research done over the past fifteen years. Knee biomechanics are more clearly understood and underlying structural/mechanical faults are recognized as initiating and then perpetuating nontraumatic knee pain.

The causative factor is weakness in a small portion of the quadriceps called the *vastus medialis obliquus* (VMO). The quadriceps is comprised of four individual muscles which work as a group. The vastus medialis is the innermost muscle, making up a portion of your inner thigh. The four muscles originate on the pelvis and combine to form the quadriceps tendon at the lower thigh; the tendon inserts on the upper end of the shin. At the lower end of the vastus medialis is a group of obliquely oriented muscle fibers, running from an upper/inner direction to a lower/outer direction. These fibers, the VMO, insert on the upper/inner half of the patella. The function of the VMO is to maintain the kneecap in a central location during extension (straightening) of the knee.

This function is critically important to effective knee mechanics. The knee has a number of variously curved, complexly oriented surfaces. There is a tendency for the kneecap to track laterally, or drift to the outer aspect of the knee, during leg extension. An intact VMO resists this lateral drift and allows flexion/extension without irritation or damage to the surrounding soft tissues. If the VMO is weak, the tendency for lateral drift of the patella will be unopposed. Since the knee bends and straightens throughout the day, chronic irritative forces are placed upon the muscular and connective tissue fibers holding the knee in position. Ultimately, this chronic irritation will cause inflammation and pain, with possible associated soft tissue injury. One structure that is specifically injured in this patellar pain syndrome is the *patellar retinaculum,* a netlike web of connective tissue fibers that support the knee joint.

Thus, the hallmark of this type of knee problem is *generalized* pain, since the injured fibers surround the knee joint. Pain is initially low-grade, only present occasionally. However, if untreated, pain increases in intensity and frequency and may become sharp. Unless a physician is consulted who has familiarity with this specific entity, the treatment or advice offered is not helpful. The person might be told, "There's no definite pathology. You just have to live with it." A diagnosis of chondromalacia might be proposed with a prescription for anti-inflammatory medication. Or quad sets might be suggested. None of this is helpful.

The answer lies in identification of the VMO weakness. This finding supports a diagnosis of *patellofemoral pain syndrome* or *extensor mechanism dysfunction,* both terms suggesting the generalized, mechanical nature of this problem. Of course, there are a lot of other problems that will result in knee pain, but those diagnoses tend to have different histories and are based on other specific findings. Patellofemoral pain syndrome is both a diagnosis of exclusion and an entity with its own specific findings, most notably VMO weakness. Effective treatment is concerned with strengthening the VMO.

VMO retraining is done lying on your back on the floor. Roll up two towels to make a roll that is four- or five-inches thick. Place that roll underneath the injured knee (Figure 10.15). The roll will collapse a little with the weight of your knee—use thick towels. You may place a few pillows underneath your head to prop it up. Now, moving your leg slowly, straighten the knee that is on the towel without pressing down on the towel and without lifting your knee off the towel (Figure 10.16).

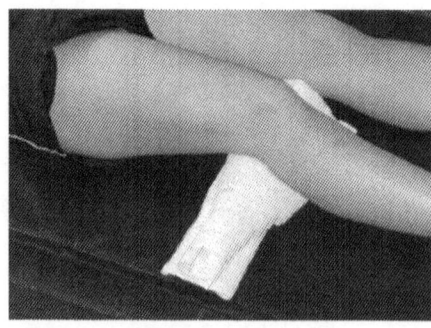

Figure 10.15

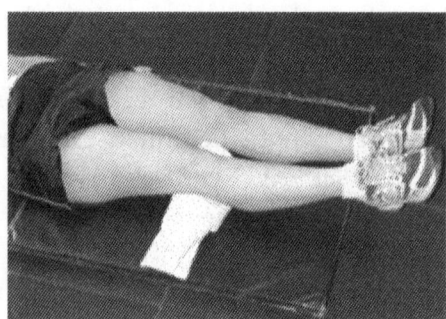

Figure 10.16

The movement itself is simple (straightening your knee), but doing it without pressing down and without lifting off is pretty challenging, particularly if your VMO is weak. This movement is called *terminal arc extension,* and involves straightening the leg the last five degrees of knee extension.

It is critical to concentrate on the VMO itself while you're straightening your leg. The VMO starts about two inches or so above the kneecap and its fibers run obliquely from the inside of the thigh down to the upper/inner half of the patella (Figure 10.17). Visualize the fibers in your mind and focus on them "working" while you slowly straighten your knee. It is both the concentration on the movement, carefully straightening without pressing down and without lifting off, and the visualization of the VMO that will retrain this small, critically important part of the quadriceps.

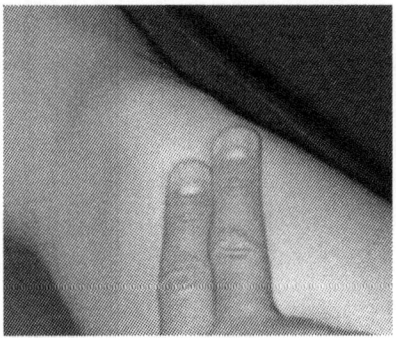

Figure 10.17

Start by doing two sets of eight reps. The movement is slow and steady, reaching through the knee into the calf, visualizing the oblique fibers of the VMO, working through those five degrees of terminal arc extension. Do the exercise four times a week and build to three sets of eight. Then you could go to a sporting goods store and purchase a Velcro ankle wrap that comes with five one-pound slugs. Each slug fits into a pocket on the ankle wrap. Wrap the little belt around your ankle, insert one of the slugs, and do two sets of six reps. Build to three sets of eight over a week or so, and then start over with two slugs. Ultimately you'll be doing three sets of eight reps with a five-pound ankle wrap. At that point your knee should be pretty well healed. I don't have experimental data to offer, but the empiric results in my office over the years suggest that nine out of ten people with generalized knee pain have very good to excellent responses to this rehabilitation program.

Lower extremity stretching is a critical part of knee rehabilitation. Hamstring, calf, and/or quadriceps tightness can create and/or perpetuate knee pain. It's good to stretch these muscle groups four or five times a week to support your VMO exercises.

As your knee pain resolves, begin aerobic exercise such as stair-climbing or running. The goal is to get back to aerobic fitness, which has been lost due to the knee problem. Start slowly, training for twelve or fifteen minutes, and build up over four weeks to thirty minutes of moderate exercise. Then you can increase the length and intensity of your workouts without being concerned about a possible relapse. Should your VMO training be ongoing? The initial phase will take, on average, three months or so. By that point you will be much improved and probably doing aerobic activity. Decrease the number of VMO sessions to twice a week, and maintain this level for two months. If knee pain returns in the future, simply go back to your VMO training, starting with a one-pound slug.

One last point to consider is knee alignment. In Chapter 4 we looked at lower extremity positioning. We talked about "straight energies", that is, having the hip socket, kneecap, and first/second toe in one straight line, rather than having lines of energy (between the hip and knee and between the knee and first/second toe) crossing at the knee. Visualizing a straight line of muscle action, from the hip to the knee and from the knee to the ankle–first/second toe, will aid in normalizing knee function and reducing pain. Think about these straight energies while you are walking, running, or climbing stairs. Your body will respond efficiently and gracefully.

Shin Splints

Shin splints is a classical overuse injury. It's a challenging injury, both in terms of accurate diagnosis and recovery. "Shin splints" is the colloquial name for a strain of the tibialis posterior, a muscle overlying the rear of the tibia (shin bone). The tibialis posterior helps to point the foot, and is active in walking, running, and jumping. Like any other muscle, the posterior tibialis can be strained by improper training techniques, doing too much too soon, or simply overtraining without sufficient rest. The person will experience a deep, dull ache or soreness along the back and inside of the shin (posteromedial pain). There may be sharp pain. Probably, the pain initially occurred toward the end of activity. If ignored, the intensity of pain will increase over subsequent training periods, until it becomes too great to continue exercising.

One challenge with shin splints is that the injury may initially appear mild. You keep going, thinking the pain will work itself out. So, shin splints often keep getting worse until you're forced to stop. Another difficulty is in obtaining a precise diagnosis. Local shin pain may actually represent a stress fracture of the tibia, brought on by the same set of conditions that would produce a tibialis posterior strain. Naturally, it's important to differentiate between these entities. The time required to heal a stress fracture is rather longer than that needed to heal a muscle strain (four to six weeks versus two to four weeks). A misdiagnosed stress fracture will worsen with improper treatment, possibly leading to long-term consequences. There is also something called *anterior compartment syndrom,e* in which swelling from an injured *tibialis anterior* causes compression of nerves and arteries in front of the shin (where there's not much room to begin with). The shin is cold, there is a loss of sensation, and the pulse is diminished or lost.

Anterior compartment syndrome is an emergency situation. Therefore, shin pain needs to be taken seriously and evaluated by an expert. Of course, most shin pain *is* caused by a tibialis posterior strain and can be diagnosed as shin splints. The area of tenderness extends for about two inches along the back and inside of the shin, right along the bone. Sometimes the pain can be reproduced by rising up on the toes or by holding the foot pointed against resistance. The pain of a tibial stress fracture is more discrete, the area of tenderness covering at the most half an inch. Percussion (tapping) over the painful area will reproduce intense local pain. Possibly, a vibrating tuning fork placed over the site will reproduce the pain. Thus, differentiating between shin splints and a tibial stress fracture is pretty clear. The physician needs to be aware of the possibility of a stress fracture and not merely write off any low-grade, nagging shin pain as shin splints.

How to treat a painful shin? For both stress fractures and shin splints, the primary form of treatment is rest. This is *relative rest,* i.e., you can continue with a cross-training form of exercise that doesn't involve repetitive motion of the lower extremity. For shin pain, weight-training is the best form of cross-training. It's important to rest the injury until the pain has completely resolved. Shin splints might heal in a week or it might take four weeks. Stress fractures will take at least four weeks to heal, probably six weeks. As usual, when the pain is gone return to activity slowly. Shin pain specifically means there's still a problem and the provocative activity will prolong the recovery period. Build back to previous levels gradually. Modify your program to eliminate the possibility of overtraining.

Two exercises for the calf, the standing toe raise for the gastrocnemius and the seated toe raise for the deeper soleus (described in Chapter 6), are very useful in preventing a return of either shin problem. Point-and-flex range-of-motion exercises for the ankle can be used as well.

Prevention lies in avoiding overtraining. We all do dumb things occasionally. We *all* do. If you notice the beginning of low-grade shin pain, take it as a warning and evaluate more closely what you've been doing. You may notice you've been doing too much, either in terms of intensity or sequence. For example, if you have a full-time job, training six days a week is usually too much. If you're twenty-four years old you might be able to pull this off, but if you're forty-four, things will definitely begin to break down. Rest days are as important as training days. Recovery time is essential to the tearing down/building up process of exercise. If you're continually in tearing-down mode, without enough rest days to maintain the building-up process, your musculoskeletal system will fail. Five days of exercise per week, interspersed with two rest days, is an appropriate maximum. Three or four days of exercise per week is realistic for most of us and completely sufficient to produce a wonderful level of fitness.

Let's look at the physiology of stress fractures. A stress fracture results from greater-than-normal stresses applied over time to *normal* bone. This is distinct from both traumatic fractures and pathological fractures. In traumatic fractures, severe acute stress is applied to a normal bone. For example, a person might be thrown from a motorcycle and fractures his thigh bone. Or, a cinder block falls on a person's foot and fractures a toe. Pathologic fractures result when normal stresses are applied to *abnormal* bone. Bone may become abnormal from a number of disease process. If the bone is a weight-bearing structure, such as the thigh bone or a lumbar vertebra, when enough of the bone has become abnormal it will fracture spontaneously, possibly during normal daily activity. In stress fractures, greater-than-normal stresses experienced on a repetitive basis cause the bone to break. Normally, bone remodels along lines of physiologic stress (Wolff's law). This means that bone will strengthen itself along lines of increased weight-bearing by building more bone to support the load.

Muscles need approximately forty-eight hours to recover from vigorous exercise. If you work muscles without allowing for sufficient rest, injury is possible because repair of damaged tissues has not been completed. Similarly, bone needs time to remodel, to strengthen itself to meet new requirements, such as running, climbing stairs, or walking longer distances. So, the bone may be normal, but it's not prepared to carry the repetitive loads because of lack of sufficient rest, and the bone fails: it breaks. Stress fractures are incomplete fractures: the fracture does not extend the full width of the bone. Also, the fracture is quite narrow in a vertical dimension. A stress fracture represents a site of failure of bony tissue. Common locations are the tibia (shin) and the second and third metatarsals, as well as the heel bone (calcaneus) and the fibula (calf bone). The pain is experienced as a deep, dull ache; variously, there may be sharp pain. Characteristically, the pain of a stress fracture is related to activity and *relieved* by rest.

Treatment for metatarsal, calcaneal, and fibular stress fractures is the same as for tibial stress fractures: rest. Do weight-training for the upper body until the fracture is healed. A "sling" may be made for an injured metatarsal by cutting out a 4-inch X 0.5-inch piece of 0.25-inch–thick adhesive foam. The foam is sticky on one surface; the molded piece is placed under the injured metatarsal to provide support during weight-bearing. After about four or five weeks of rest, try to run a little. If there's no pain, the next day run a little more. If there's still no pain, the stress fracture has healed and you can *slowly* return to aerobic training.

Ankle Sprains

One of the challenges with ankle sprains is that once you've injured an ankle, it seems so easy to re-injure it. I've heard many dancers say, "Oh, I injured my ankle and you know, you never get over it. You're never the same after an ankle sprain." Other people report, "I have weak ankles. I've had many ankle sprains." It's often the case that a single ankle sprain turns into a recurring injury—however, this scenario represents a failure of appropriate treatment. With effective acute management and systematic, simple rehabilitation, an ankle injury can remain a one-time event.

OK. You're walking along and if you're a New Yorker, chances are that one day you'll step into a crack in the sidewalk and twist your ankle. Or in another scenario, you're ice skating, you catch an edge, and your ankle turns over. Or you're playing volleyball, you're at the net, you jump high to spike the ball and land with your foot on top of your unsuspecting teammate's foot, and you badly twist your ankle, as I did one summer at the beach. Your ankle swells a little, within two hours it's a little blue, and it really hurts to put weight on it so you're limping. There might be a lot of swelling and a lot of blue discoloration. Severe pain would suggest a complete tear of one or more of the ankle ligaments. In any case, regardless of what you think about the injury, my suggestion is to have your ankle sprain evaluated by your sports physician.

The initial treatment is the same for all ankle sprains, whether mild, moderate, or severe: rest, ice, compression, and elevation. We discussed this RICE protocol earlier in this chapter; all elements apply to acute ankle sprains. Rest is relative rest. An Aircast® ankle brace allows you to walk while taking the weight-bearing load off the injured ligaments. Be sure to use ice frequently, apply an ankle wrap when the brace is off, and elevate your leg whenever and wherever possible. Elevation reduces swelling and pain by creating a gravity gradient, draining the excess fluid into the venous and lymphatic systems. It's important to reduce this local fluid accumulation for several reasons, not the least of which is to avoid perpetuating an inflammatory reaction. When using ice, wrap the cold pack in a towel and apply it for fifteen minutes every two hours. Apply ice about four times a day for about three days.

Depending on the extent of the injury, it might take two weeks or more for the swelling to completely resolve. During this time the discoloration will shift from blue to yellow-green to brown as the hemoglobin in the pooled blood is metabolized. If you're wearing an Aircast® brace, you could keep in shape by doing weight-training routines for your upper body, obtaining a cross-training effect for your leg muscles. When the swelling is mostly gone and pain levels are mild, you can begin a rehabilitation program that will help prevent ankle sprains in the future.

We're looking to create "smart" ankles in this rehabilitation program. Sprains, by definition, are injuries to ligaments—ligamentous fibers are torn and neurologic connections between the ligaments and the brain are disrupted. Of particular importance in the ankle is loss of *proprioceptor* function. Proprioceptors are nerve cells that provide information about the body's position in space. The ankle is just about where the rubber meets the road. The entire weight of the body is transmitted through the ankle to the foot to the floor, and ankle integrity is critical to normal walking, running, and jumping. Diminished proprioception makes the ankle floppy: the foot doesn't quite know where it is, adaptations to variations in ground surface aren't quite as instantaneous, and the actions of placing the foot on the ground and lifting it off are less than perfect.

The lack of rehabilitation of proprioception explains why one ankle sprain is frequently followed by others; it explains why people develop "weak" ankles after an ankle sprain. The ankles are weak because they're "dumber" than they were before the initial injury. Computing power has been lost and there are glitches in the instantaneous calculations necessary to maintain smooth, effortless function. These ankles turn over and twist easily, and the person suffers repeated low-grade injuries or worse. The key to successful rehabilitation is to establish new and better proprioceptive linkages. This is easily done by utilizing a few simple techniques.

One exercise is *toe gripping*. In a seated position, place both bare feet flat on the floor. Grip the toes, clenching them hard so the arch of your foot comes off the floor, hold for a few seconds, and relax. Do this ten times. Another exercise is to place the injured ankle in a bucket of warm water, and "write" the letters of the alphabet with your foot. This is more difficult than it sounds and provides great practice in ankle coordination. You could "write" capital letters one day and lower case letters the next.

A third exercise is resisted ankle pointing (plantarflexion) and flexing (dorsiflexion) with a Thera-Band®. For plantarflexion, place the Thera-Band® around the ball of your foot, like a sling, and hold the other end in your hand. Place tension on the Thera-Band® by pulling on it, and point your foot against the resistance. Do this ten times. An assistant is needed to do dorsiflexion. The Thera-Band® is placed over the top of your foot and your assistant holds the ends, placing tension on the Thera-Band®. Dorsiflex your foot against the resistance. Repeat for a set of ten. You could do two total sets (pointing and flexing) each day.

Next is what could be termed the "flamingo" or "stork" exercise, because the exercise position resembles that of familiar shore birds, who of course have *terrific* proprioception. This simple, yet challenging, routine provides specific rehabilitation for ankle proprioceptors. Let's say you injured your right ankle. You stand a little less than arm's length from a wall, with your right arm perpendicular to the wall, and lightly touch the wall with the fingers of your right hand. This will prevent you from toppling over if you lose your balance. Stand on the right leg and place the left foot beside the right knee, so that the left knee is bent and facing directly front (Figure 10.18). Maintain this position for about twenty seconds, balancing on the right leg. Your right ankle will wobble a little as it readjusts to stabilize your weight. These oscillations will continue for the duration of the exercise; they represent your proprioceptive system in a dynamic, learning state. Early on, you might lose your balance every so often; that's part of the training. You're reestablishing a connection between your brain and the structures of the ankle joint. You're relearning how to achieve and maintain balance so that walking, running, and jumping become smooth, coordinated activities.

OK, you've done the right leg. Turn around and do the same thing on the left (uninjured leg). Now, go back to the right leg, but this time, after you've placed the left foot at the right knee, turn out the left leg so the left knee is facing to the side—this would be called a passé position in ballet (Figure 10.19).

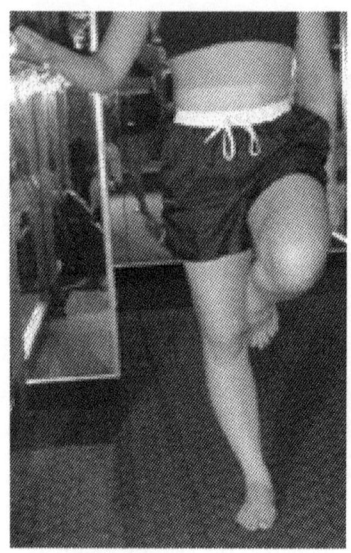 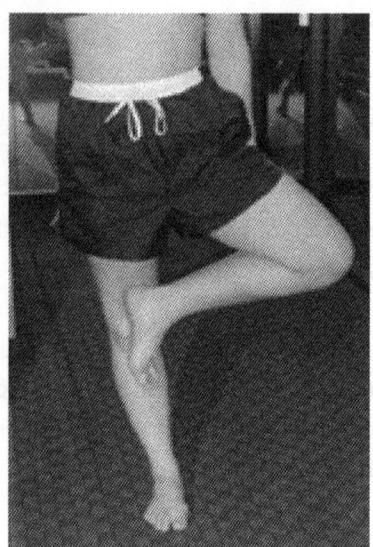

Figure 10.18   Figure 10.19

Maintain this balanced position for twenty seconds and then do the same thing standing on the left leg. Thus, the whole routine is right leg, left leg, with the opposite knee facing front; right leg, left leg, with the opposite knee turned out. That's it. Do the whole routine twice a day, and after a month both ankles will be very smart.

Typically, the result will be ankles that are strong and do not re-injure. Your ankle will still turn over occasionally—there are drastically uneven surfaces out there. You might even stumble and twist an ankle. But owing to the increased "smartness" of your ankles, the ligaments and muscle-tendon units will adapt to possible extreme stresses without tearing of fibers. Occasionally, in the last few years, I have severely turned over each of my ankles without any lasting pain. Each time I thought, "oh, no, not another ankle sprain". But I've been fine, without a hint of swelling or pain. This result derives from effective rehabilitation of the ankle sprains I did have. The time involved in doing the rehabilitative exercises is well spent.

Overuse Syndromes

It seems that the incidence of overuse syndromes has increased exponentially over the last ten years. The most commonly diagnosed of these conditions is carpal tunnel syndrome. Painful overuse syndromes of the elbow and shoulder are also common. I propose that carpal tunnel syndrome is overdiagnosed and many, if not most, of these diagnoses are inaccurate. If treatment of the painful wrist and/or hand fails, surgery to release the carpal tunnel may be recommended. This is unfortunate, as successful outcomes for this type of surgery are not frequently obtained. Surgical outcomes have been less than satisfactory because the initial diagnoses were in error. Actual, verifiable carpal tunnel syndrome may need surgical decompression if conservative treatment fails. My point is that most wrist/hand overuse syndromes are *not* carpal tunnel syndrome.

The carpal tunnel lies between the palmar surface of the wrist bones and the transverse carpal ligament. A person with carpal tunnel syndrome experiences numbness and/or tingling in the thumb and second and third fingers; numbness may involve the entire hand. Pain may be felt in the same location. Pain is characteristically *paroxysmal* in nature, that is, spasmodic, occurring as a sudden attack, frequently awakening a person from sleep. There may be pain on the outside of the forearm, as well. Pain in the wrist is *not* a typical symptom of carpal tunnel syndrome. Carpal tunnel syndrome may be associated with pregnancy, rheumatoid arthritis, osteoarthritis, and trauma, all of which may cause narrowing of the carpal tunnel.

If you don't have these particular symptoms, you don't have spasmodic, paroxysmal pain, you don't have pain that wakes you up at night, but *do* have generalized wrist and hand pain, you probably don't have carpal tunnel syndrome. What do you have, then? Most probably, a *scleratogenous* pain syndrome, related to irritation of muscles, tendons, ligaments, and joints. The *scleratome* is the portion of an embryo from which bone, ligament, muscle, and tendon develop. Scleratogenous pain is local or radiating pain, caused by irritation of any or several of these tissues. Such irritation can result from repetitive use, particularly, repetitive use in biomechanically inefficient positions. Let's say you do a lot of work at a computer. Your keyboard might be too low or too high. Your monitor might be too high or placed at an angle to your keyboard, so you have to rotate your head to see it. The only free space for your computer mouse might be up on a shelf or across the desk. Your chairback might be too stiff, or your chair might be too low or too high.

In any of these situations, eventually you may develop arm-related pain. Your wrist begins to hurt, or your fingers and/or hand begin to feel achy and stiff. You may begin to experience elbow and/or forearm pain. Pain is probably more intense at night. This is not because you have carpal tunnel syndrome, but relates to the fact that you've worked all day and irritated the joints and soft tissues of your arm.

This particular set of symptoms is very discouraging. The low-grade pain may be continuous, may be worsening, and becomes an annoyance that interferes with the quality of your life. Acute pain can be treated, but there doesn't seem to be any prospect of improvement for an upper extremity overuse syndrome. In fact, there *are* a number of steps that can be taken, both at the workplace and in the activities of daily living. First and foremost, ergonomic solutions regarding your computer set-up are required. According to *The New Oxford Shorter English Dictionary*, ergonomics is "the field of study that deals with the relationship between people and their working environment, as it affects efficiency, safety, and ease of action". Ergonomic evaluation of computer work-stations has led to a number of recommendations:

- The chair seat height should be aligned with the keyboard, so that when the person's hands are on the keyboard, his elbows are parallel to the floor. In other words, in an ergonomically efficient typing position, the elbows are neither above nor below the level of the keyboard.

- Similarly, the mouse should be immediately adjacent to the keyboard, so that good elbow alignment is maintained.
- The monitor should be placed so that the person's neck flexes slightly and the person's angle of gaze is directed downward about ten degrees. Looking up engages neck and upper back muscles, leading to muscle tightness and fatigue. Looking down at a slight angle alleviates this unnecessary tension. Rotating the head to look at the monitor is a gross violation of ergonomic principles.
- The monitor display should be crisp and clear.
- It is useful to get up every half hour or so and take a quick break, possibly getting a brief change of scenery and some fresh air.

There are clinical solutions as well. Chiropractic manipulation of the neck and upper back may provide benefit. There will almost always be associated trigger points of the trapezius and rhomboid musculature. Such trigger points can themselves be responsible for radiating arm pain, and treatment will reduce pain levels.

Active care involves postural considerations and exercise. You knew there would be exercise in this somewhere, right? The most important postural recommendation is to let the shoulder girdle rest on the rib cage. Shoulders tend to ride upward during the course of a workday, if you're not paying attention to your posture. This persistent muscular contraction wastes energy, creates fatigue, and ultimately produces trigger points which cause pain. Shoulder, elbow, and wrist joints participate in this cycle of tension. Gently remind yourself to let go of these tight neck and upper back muscles, allowing the shoulders to assume a neutral position and rest on the upper rib cage.

Any exercise will help, particularly if you haven't exercised in a long while. Start walking for exercise, and build up to 30 minutes or more of brisk activity. Buy a set of light dumbbells and begin the upper body workouts described in Chapter 6. Exercise will reduce stress, lengthen short muscles, promote circulation, and increase your well-being. Each of these elements will help reduce the pain of a wrist/hand overuse syndrome.

Thus, the solution to this difficult problem is fourfold: ergonomic considerations, joint manipulative therapy, postural improvement, and exercise. Typically, improvement is gradual and steady. In the best scenario, the problem is recognized early and intervention is immediate. Naturally, daily, chronic pain will take longer to resolve. As long as there continues to be noticeable improvement, however little, the recovery is progressing well.

Muscle Strains

We've all had muscle strains and we're going to have more of them. This is the nature of training (and life). Being fit and engaged in the path of fitness certainly reduces the incidence of injuries and significantly improves one's recovery time from injuries. But breakdowns occur. What are you going to do about it and how are you going to get better? The main principle, as we've seen before, is *relative rest*. Rest the injured muscle and train everything else, applying the related principle of cross-training. Here's one basic guideline—if it hurts, don't do it.

Now, you want to be cautious, but not over-cautious. Being over-cautious might delay your recovery unnecessarily, but not being cautious enough might lead to re-injury. It's a fine line. Basically, if you've strained a muscle, for example, your calf or quadriceps, resting that muscle for one week is a good minimum. Anything less than one week is probably not sufficient for healing. More extensive injuries require more rest; this is simply common sense. It's important to admit the existence of the injury and allow the time needed for recovery. Denial will perpetuate the problem. You do some routine you're not ready for, and now you're two steps backward, rather than making stepwise progress. Your sports physician is an expert resource in judging the extent of an injury and the likely time needed for rest.

I prefer to err on the side of activity, but only after there has been a period of rest and pain levels have reduced. If it still hurts to walk, obviously you can't run. Timing the return to activity is not a science, it's instinctual based on experience, and there are a number of variables to consider. For example, I recently treated Richard, the president of a consumer products company. I've helped him for many years for various back-related complaints, and he was in my office because of a mild, but annoying, sacroiliac sprain. He was much better after two visits, still had some low-grade discomfort, and wanted to know if he could play in his family's annual Thanksgiving touch football game.

My first thought was, no, that could be a problem, but after reflecting for a minute and considering the *life* variables, I concluded Richard wanted to play and was asking for my assurance that it would *be* OK. Richard is in great shape, he's always maintained a full exercise program, and he's mentally tough. I said, yes, you can play, and if you're a little worse afterward, we'll pick up the pieces next week. Really, what were the possible consequences? If it was a tackle game, I would have recommended against it. It was a family event, and it sounded like a lot of fun. Did it really matter if he came out of it a little worse for a few days? We agreed that it wouldn't matter. It was a risk we agreed it would be OK to take.

On the other hand, another recent patient, Jeanne, had lower back pain with radiating pain into her right buttock and around the front of her right thigh. The radiating pain was described as burning in nature. This was probably more than a muscle/ligament strain/sprain, and her examination suggested that a mass lesion was causing her symptoms. The most likely diagnosis was a herniated disc, and I referred her for magnetic resonance imaging. A small disc herniation was identified which was irritating a spinal nerve root. She began a course of anti-inflammatory medication and gentle spinal manipulation. After a few days she was feeling better, and wanted to know when she could go back to exercise.

Jeanne is a nurse at a local hospital and is in good shape—she does aerobics and lifts weights regularly. With Jeanne, however, it was necessary to return to exercise *gradually*. Too much activity would exacerbate her problem, which was just beginning to resolve. A good approach involved stretches for her hamstrings, calves, and quadriceps and some mild activity on a stationary bike. Jeanne continued to improve over several weeks, and then returned to a step aerobics class and lifting light weights. Her radiating pain pattern resolved in two weeks.

People also seek treatment for neck pain and back pain, acute or chronic. These are people who work hard, have families, and generally are not inclined to exercise, never liked it, or used to be in shape and believe they have too many other responsibilities and no time to exercise. But now, at the end of the consultation/examination, a person might say, "What exercises should I be doing?" Or, "Can I go to the gym in a couple of days?" Well, not only will exercise not *cure* acute pain, it will make you worse. Exercise is not *treatment*.

These mechanical back problems are directly related, to a large extent, to deconditioning, but *reconditioning* is not part of the first phase of recovery. I reply, "Great. It's good that you want to begin exercising, but it's not time yet to do that." Instead, I prescribe lower extremity stretches or neck/upper back stretches. As pain resolves, in a week or two, mild exercises are started. Exercise intensity increases over time. One main point is that exercise is not a panacea and is definitely not a *short-term* solution. The equation, "I have back pain; I should exercise" is inaccurate and a little dangerous. Here's a more effective approach: "I have back pain, and probably one of the causes is that I haven't exercised in a long time. I will learn how to recover properly and start a good, comprehensive exercise program when I am able." This works.

The timeline and sequencing of return to activity needs to be individualized. Strict "rules" are inappropriate. A professional dancer, a computer programmer who plays in a competitive volleyball league, and a securities analyst who hasn't exercised since high school have widely differing needs and goals. An astute physician recognizes and addresses these differences, designing his recommendations for the individual. It is necessary, though, for the *context* of treatment to be *return to activity.*

Hamstring Strains

Hamstring strains are common in sports. We frequently hear about this professional football player or that star college basketball player who has injured a hamstring and is out of action for at least a month. To be *hamstrung* implies that your efficiency is hindered; a hamstrung person is *frustrated.* I can attest to the frustration inherent in a hamstring strain, having had three separate hamstring injuries when I was dancing. There's not a lot to do for such an injury. If you're a professional athlete, you might walk around with an electrical stimulator strapped to your thigh, but most of us won't be doing that. Thigh wraps have been fashionable in the NBA for the last few years, with the hope of keeping the thigh muscles warm and thus avoiding injury.

Hamstring injuries are difficult to heal completely. An injury at the origin of the muscle group, the ischial tuberosity, will take a long time to heal, anywhere from six to twelve months. If lifting your leg and trying to straighten your knee produces pain underneath your buttock at the top of your thigh, you've strained the origin of the hamstrings. A hamstring injury can occur in the belly (middle) of the hamstring group. The pain of a mid-hamstring injury is felt in the middle portion of the thigh. Mid-hamstring strains will heal more rapidly, possibly within four to six weeks.

A hamstring strain may result from poor technique, overexertion, or simply playing hard and making a sudden, short stop. Tight muscles lead to muscle/tendon injuries. If you are physically active, it's a good idea to consistently stretch your lower back and leg muscles. Also, inefficient pelvic biomechanics can cause hamstring strains. If the sacroiliac joints are not achieving their full range of motion, the hamstrings may tighten to compensate for the altered load-bearing. Over time the muscles will fatigue and fail.

Treatment consists of ice applications for the first 72 hours postinjury, elevation if the injury is severe, and relative rest. Hamstring recovery is slow because these muscles are used in most activities of daily living. Do your best to avoid activities that make it hurt. However, after a couple of weeks of resting from your particular sport, you may start to return to activity. The timing will vary depending on the severity of the injury (for example, visible discoloration in the mid-thigh is evidence of a severe strain), but most hamstring strains are mild to moderate. Such a hamstring strain is one of the few injuries that it makes sense to *work through*. We've all heard this term: *work through* your injury. How do you go about doing this and actually get better? What does it mean to work through an injury?

Working Through an Injury

Well, most injuries should not be "worked through". If you try to keep going, you'll simply increase the severity of the injury and prolong or even prevent recovery. You can't work through shin splints, stress fractures, or ankle sprains. You can't work through a tennis elbow or a rotator cuff strain. As we've discussed, recovery from these injuries requires specific rehabilitation. However, an injury to large, bulky muscles, such as the hamstrings and quadriceps, can be worked through after a short period of rest, possibly one or two weeks. Most mild (possibly even moderate) strain/sprain injuries to the neck and back can be worked through. Rib muscle strains can be worked through.

You can work through an injury when additional rest will not have a significant impact on the rate of recovery. Implicit in working through is the concept that activity will not cause a setback. So, working through an injury does not mean being foolish. It means going back to the gym, the track, the tennis court, or dance class and doing those things, but on a diminished level initially. It also means being careful to avoid any activity that causes *sharp* pain. Sharp pain denotes tearing of muscle fibers. If you have sharp pain, you're doing too much; reducing the intensity should cause the sharp pain to disappear. If it persists, stop exercising, and rest again for several days before returning to activity. Proceed carefully when working through an injury. There will be achy or dull pain, possibly tightness or stiffness. Everything's fine, provided these sensations are low-grade. Throbbing pain at the end of the day means you did too much. Do less the next time.

There are some caveats to this process of working through. It's easier to work through an injury if you're already in good shape. If you weren't in such good condition when you got hurt, allow more time to heal before returning to activity. Also, working through implies you know what you're doing. If you're a beginner, have your sports physician guide you through the process of recovery, regardless.

Now, really, how can you work through an injury? The method includes warming up effectively, employing careful and strict technique, and "listening" to your body. By avoiding sharp pain, you're not creating further damage, and exercise actually provides therapy in the form of increased local metabolism. More oxygen and other nutrients are brought to the muscle than when the muscle is resting, and metabolic end-products of the tissue reparative process are removed more efficiently. In cases when working through an injury is appropriate, activity actually *speeds* recovery. Rest is needed in the short term. A long-term recommendation of rest should always be questioned. For example, in the case of a hamstring strain at its origin, dull pain and restricted mobility will not completely resolve for many months, possibly a year. Is rest needed until the pain is gone? No. Is activity necessary to maintain conditioning and fitness while the injury is healing? Yes. Herein lies the concept of working through an injury.

Disc Herniations

Disc herniations are a challenging problem, both for the physician and the patient. Modern imaging methods, computed tomography ("CAT scan") and magnetic resonance imaging (MRI) have uncovered many disc herniations that would otherwise have gone undetected. These techniques are immensely valuable, but they have also created diagnostic dilemmas. Many of the herniations discovered are not related to the person's problem. Current medical literature suggests that at least 20% of normal persons have a herniated disc. It is possible to have low back pain and also have a lumbar herniated disc that is unrelated to the pain. It's an error to conclude that the disc herniation seen on an imaging study is necessarily the cause of the pain. Various commissions have developed criteria by which a clinical correlation can be made, enabling a physician to state with a high degree of certainty that the disc herniation is related to the pain.

These criteria need to be met to conclude that such a causative relationship exists. Criteria exist for evaluating both the clinical status of the patient and the findings on the imaging study. If both sets of criteria are satisfied, a causal relationship can be inferred. Disc herniations that actually contact a spinal nerve, causing an inflammatory response that involves radiating pain into the forearm/hand or calf/foot, are certainly more challenging to treat than joint-related pain that radiates into an extremity. Still, the large majority of these disc herniations can be successfully treated (very good to excellent results) with conservative methods. Statistically, only between five and ten percent of disc herniations require surgical intervention.

Let's consider lower back pain associated with lower extremity pain, and contrast joint-related symptoms versus leg pain related to a symptomatic herniated disc. In the first case, lower back pain is the predominant symptom. There may be pain radiating into the buttock and thigh, possibly into the calf, and you think, or have been told, that you have "sciatica". Sciatica refers to inflammation of the sciatic nerve, a thick nerve that traverses the piriformis muscle, exits the pelvis, and innervates the thigh, calf, and foot. Symptoms include radiating leg pain into the foot, and possibly numbness or a pins-and-needles sensation radiating into the foot.

Sciatica is caused by a variety of conditions; in itself, "sciatica" describes the radiating lower extremity sensations. It's not an effective diagnostic term. Possible causes of sciatic nerve pain include diabetes, alcoholism, local bone infection, disease of a vertebra (tumor or infection), hip dislocation, arthritis, disc herniation, and lower back strain/sprain injuries. Thus, leg pain associated with back pain needs to be taken seriously and evaluated thoroughly, not merely written off as "sciatica". Fortunately, in the large majority of cases, leg pain that accompanies a primary complaint of lower back pain represents a reflex response to the lower back soft tissue injury. In such cases, lower extremity pain represents referred *scleratogenous* pain, that is, referred pain from injured joints, ligaments, and muscle/tendon units.

Your sports physician evaluates your back pain which is accompanied by lower extremity pain. He rules out the disease-related causes and concludes the leg pain is not "sciatica", but rather scleratogenous referred pain from the lower back. You proceed accordingly, treat as necessary, do rehabilitation exercises as described above for strain/sprains, and recover.

In the second scenario, radiating pain into the calf and/or foot is the primary symptom. There may be lower back pain but it is not the chief complaint. There may be numbness and tingling or pins-and-needles sensations radiating into the calf and/or foot. Coughing, sneezing, or straining will exacerbate the radiating pain or numbness. Certain maneuvers your doctor performs elicit or exacerbate the lower extremity sensations. In sum, this scenario represents an inflamed spinal nerve root. The cause is a mass pressing on the nerve root. The most likely mass is a herniated disc, specifically diagnosed with magnetic resonance imaging.

OK, you have a herniated disc. Now what? Ice applications for fifteen minutes every two hours act as a sedative, decreasing pain. Rest is useful for a few days while the initial inflammation subsides. Anti-inflammatory medication reduces the irritation and swelling of the nerve root, and aids in removal of metabolic end-products that may perpetuate the inflammation. Over-the-counter anti-inflammatory medication may be sufficient, but often stronger, prescription-only medication is needed. Joint mobilization and/or manipulation may be helpful in restoring more normal biomechanics and in reducing pain through the gating control mechanism.

These therapeutic measures are directed toward the acute injury; symptoms will typically resolve within two to six weeks. There should be a steady, noticeable improvement over this period. For the minority of cases that do not resolve, surgery may be an appropriate solution, depending on the circumstances. Let's discuss rehabilitation for the majority of disc injuries in which most of the symptoms resolve satisfactorily.

These basic recommendations are intended to be considered in the context of a particular case. Some persons will be able to do and achieve more, others less. As always, the first consideration is your overall level of fitness. If extra weight is a factor, a graduated weight-reduction program is necessary. Let the weight loss be a *self-expression,* rather than something you *have to do.* Lose weight slowly and steadily, setting realistic targets. Losing ten pounds in six weeks is realistic and doable. Next, plan to lose another ten pounds in another six weeks. Now, you've lost twenty pounds in three months, and if more is needed, you've got a proven track record and experience to guide you. If you're relatively deconditioned, you'll follow the return-to-activity protocol outlined earlier. Start by walking, build up to one-half hour of brisk walking, then go to the gym and start using a stair-climbing machine and/or riding a stationary bike. Begin by spending fifteen minutes on an aerobic-exercise machine, at a light level, and build up to one-half hour of moderately intense work. Make sure you're doing the lower extremity stretches we described in Chapter 5. Once you've obtained a good degree of aerobic fitness, it's time to begin weight-training, abdominal strengthening, and lower back exercises. We've thoroughly outlined these programs in Chapter 6. They are well-designed to support rehabilitation of a disc herniation.

Progress should be slow and steady. Any return of radiating leg pain is a specific warning that you're doing too much. It's worse to do too much rather than too little. You are training to prevent a return of the problem, not to cause a new problem. Caution is indicated, as is attention to proper alignment and technique.

If you're already fit and returning to activity after experiencing a symptomatic disc herniation, the challenge is to avoid doing too much too soon. You're finally feeling good, you want to get moving, you remember all the things you used to do, you've got the go-ahead to start, and what are you faced with? Lifting pretty light weights and running nowhere near as fast or as hard as you used to. You're way behind your personal curve. Well, OK, but really, so what? You had a significant problem and you *didn't* need surgery. So, things may be a little boring at first, but if you continue steadily you'll get progressively stronger faster. You do not want a setback here. Setbacks are troublesome, since a new inflammation implies being off activity for at least a week. You avoid this by being careful, proceeding slowly and incrementally.

What kinds of things are you doing? Light running, starting with fifteen minutes the first few times, making sure that everything is fine and building from there. Light weights, probably about one-third to one-half as heavy as you used to lift, building from there.

What kinds of things should a person who has had a symptomatic disc herniation *not* be doing? Well, you're not the person who should be lifting the air conditioner or the TV. You're not the one to be opening the very stuck window. You will always need to be careful about bending and lifting. One good principle to follow is never lift anything when you're bent over and twisted to one side. This combination of forward bending (flexion) and twisting (axial torsion) places the disc in its most mechanically compromised position. So, this position is to be avoided. In general, when lifting an object, bend your knees, activate your abdominal muscles, and be sure to hold the object close to your torso. Bending your knees prevents you from flexing too far forward at the waist when lifting something, thus avoiding extreme stresses on the spine. Active abdominal muscles will support most of the load, rather than having the load solely carried by the muscles and ligaments (including the discs) of the lumbar spine. Holding the object close to your torso significantly reduces the forces on the lumbar spine, shortening the *lever arm* between your body's long axis and the weight you're lifting.

If you follow these mechanical guidelines you will be able to bend and lift successfully, without straining your back or re-injuring the disc. However, my recommendation is to avoid heavy lifting. What if you have young kids or nieces or nephews? Do your best to be sensible. Your conditioning program *should* prevent serious re-injury. The combination of stretching, weight-training, abdominal exercise, and lower back exercise is designed to enable the lower back to support mechanical loads. A twenty-four-pound two-year-old is certainly that. Make sure you lift correctly, never lift a kid when your knees are straight, and you'll be able to have plenty of fun. And, it's useful to remember that stuff happens. Kids will jump on your back, or push or pull you unexpectedly. Your high level of conditioning, obtained by consistent training over the long term, will tend to minimize the damage of any new strain/sprain.

Coming Back Stronger

Coming back stronger is a wonderful philosophy and can become a practical reality. This principle or attitude is applicable to the events of one's life, as well as to the specific circumstances of recovering from a physical injury. With regard to the physical, usually we think an injury will cause some permanent limitation of function, of greater or lesser degree. An injury, regardless of the extent of healing, produces an area of weakness. We hear these things: "Oh, I have a bad back", or "I never fully recovered from that shoulder injury", or "I have a weak ankle". These statements may be accurate, relatively, and reflect ineffective rehabilitation strategies. Often, there has been no attempt at systematic rehabilitation. Thus, the injured region never does return to normal.

Physiologically, tissue injury involves disruption of local capillaries. Biochemical signals are distributed through the bloodstream, initiating a cascade of reparative responses. Various inflammatory cells migrate to the region of injury: these cells clean up debris, minimize further damage, and begin to repair injured structures. Fibroblasts are the cells which act as building blocks. A fibroblast has the potential to become any type of connective tissue cell: a blood cell, a cell lining a capillary wall, a bone cell, a cartilage cell, a cell in a ligament, or a cell in a tendon.

Fibroblasts are known as *primitive* cells: they are *undifferentiated* connective tissue cells and are able to differentiate into specific cell types whenever and wherever necessary. Fibroblasts will make new cells and knit together the torn edges of tendons and ligaments. Old, damaged structures are replaced by new tissue. The downside of this miraculous reparative capability is that the orientation of the new fibers is disorganized. Rather than being oriented parallel to the long axis of muscular contraction or mechanical load deformation, new connective tissue fibers are oriented randomly. If systematic rehabilitation is not done, the random orientation persists and creates a permanent area of weakness.

Thus, rehabilitation is critical to regaining normal function. What about "coming back stronger"? Except in cases of major trauma involving significant external forces, an injury highlights an area of relative weakness. An injury says, here's a region that's not strong enough or prepared enough to withstand serious work. Or, an injury might imply a technique problem, in which faulty technique creates harmful stresses on muscles, tendons, ligaments, and cartilage. You can survive faulty technique for a period of time, and then the system will fail. In the rehabilitative process both weaknesses and technique anomalies are addressed. It becomes important to pay attention to good technique, whereas previously you might have been able to get away with inaccuracies in form. Then an injury occurred. In rehabilitation, if your technique is off you'll have discomfort or pain.

It's an immediate feedback system, and your technique will necessarily become more efficient. Regarding weakness and imbalance, rehabilitation consists of specific exercises targeted to a particular region. This directed activity usually fills an unrecognized gap in a person's training, bringing an area of hidden weakness up to the fitness level of the rest of the body. Overall, you become stronger than before the injury, weak areas undergo training with intensity, and technique is optimized. You come back stronger. In general, you train with more intensity, your technique is rigorous, and your workouts are broader in focus. Coming back stronger is thus the unexpected benefit of injury.

Coming back stronger provides other intangible benefits. You have won at something important: you've been injured and come back, with discipline and focus, rather than quitting and moving on to something else. You've demonstrated the ability to get the job done, to follow through, in an unaccustomed area—your health and well-being. You've taken on adverse conditions and been willing to be patient, accepting small gains achieved over time, laying a new foundation and building a structure that will last. I recognize the hard work. I applaud the effort and the commitment.

Final Thoughts

Fitness is a journey. Fitness ebbs and flows; there are peaks and valleys. You can be in a good groove for a while, and then you have an injury and have to change your routine. That's all right. Injuries happen. What counts, most of all, is to keep going.

There is a momentum to fitness. When you haven't exercised in a while, it's easy not to exercise. But when you're in the habit of exercising, when you're used to doing it, it's easy to do. Your body pulls you along. It's instinctive.

What does it mean to be fit? For me, fitness is a metaphor. One is not only physically fit, but fit in all aspects of life. Of course, the achievement of fitness is ongoing. It's a daily discipline, one that is life-giving and life-affirming.

Thank you for spending time with me. May you be healthy and well, and may you continue to dream, fulfill your dreams, and prosper.

About the Author

▼

Dr. David Lemberg has been practicing chiropractic for twenty years, specializing in spinal conditions and sports-related injuries. He is a member of the postgraduate faculty of Los Angeles College of Chiropractic, an entity of The Southern California University of Health Sciences. For the last ten years he has taught orthopedics to chiropractors in venues across the United States and in Canada.

Dr. Lemberg was a professional dancer in his first career, studying, performing, and teaching dance in and around New York City. His interests include public speaking, photography, and computers. A new novel is in the works.